Seniors Stay Forever Young

Reclaim your life and wellness with Exercise

By

Author Norma Jean

&

Co Author Joycelyn Scott- CanFitPro FIS, PTS

Edited by Juel Gulab-Monteiro BA, MA

Seniors Stay Forever Young

Printed in Canada

Publisher: Norma Gangaram

Registration No. **1079262**

ISBN 978-0-9809499-6-4

Dedicated to:

The Mayor of Brampton, Susan Fennell, for making Flower City Seniors Recreations Centre available to all seniors of Brampton. It is also a great social environment for all seniors. Thank you!

To Sharon Bonello and her staff and instructors at Flower City and their commitment and dedication to wonderful programmes as well as their willingness to embrace new ideas such as Saturday night dance live.

To all the seniors that attend this centre who have touched my life in such a positive way and have so willingly allow me to use their pictures for this book. You are a wonderful group of people with so much to offer. I am truly blessed to have gotten to know all of you. Exercise and Stay forever young.

This book belongs to _____

Date: _____

If you borrowed this book and you enjoyed it,
I invite you to purchase your own copy at
http://www.childrensstories.ca

Acknowledgements

Thanks to my husband Rolland, who is a very private person, thank you for allowing me to put your picture on the cover of this book. Grandpa is holding our handsome grandson.

It would be impossible to express enough of my sincere gratitude to Joycelyn Scott, who so very graciously helped me with this book by lending me her expertise in fitness and instruction and, for all of her dedications in helping to make this book possible. Thank you for believing in me and standing with me on this project.

To Linda Jeffery, my yoga instructor I would like to thank you for the input and advice on the yoga section of this book, I am truly grateful. Thank you for your friendship and support.

To Carmelina Oppedisano, I would like to thank you for planting the idea of this book in my head and for believing in me to be able to write this book.

To my niece, Juel Gulab-Monteiro thank you for taking the time out of your busy schedule to edit this book so willingly and quickly.

To all the seniors who so very generously agreed to let me take their pictures for this book, thank you so very much for your support. The seniors of Brampton Flower city are a wonderful group of men and women, and I am grateful to have met all of you and have you touch my life in such a positive way. Thank you for your support.

Editor's Note

I truly believe that it is never too late to reclaim our health and well-being. A lot of times, people do not know where to start. They know that they want to exercise but they lack knowledge on available programs. This book most definitely addresses the options that currently exist. A detailed description of the various programs is clearly explained.

As an educator, I believe that this book has real-life application in the classroom as well. In physical education classes, more time is spent on active participation. Although it is crucial for young people and children alike to be active, it is important that these future citizens are aware of existing programs as they will not be in a classroom for the rest of their lives. Their knowledge of available programs and options can also inspire their grandparents and parents to become active.

In my opinion, this book is an essential piece of literature for all seniors and anyone else who enjoys fitness. The various municipalities would benefit from this book if it were available. I believe that more seniors would want to participate in recreation programs as this book helps to respond to their needs and concerns. If retirement residences incorporated this book into their programs, I believe that they would also see an increase in their number of participants involved with fitness classes.

Table of Contents   **Page**

Great Truths about Growing Old

1. Growing old is mandatory; growing up is optional.

2. Forget health food. I need all the preservatives I can get.

3. When you fall down, you wonder what else you can do while you're down there.

4. You're getting old when you get the same sensation from a rocking chair that you once got from a roller coaster.

5. It is frustrating when you know all the answers but nobody bothers to ask you the questions.

6. Time may be a great healer, but it's a lousy beautician.

7. Wisdom comes with age, but sometimes age comes alone.

Between 1981 and 2009, fitness levels of Canadian adults declined significantly, according to the first findings from the Canadian Health Measures Survey (CHMS). This is the most comprehensive national survey ever conducted in Canada to determine fitness levels.

Seniors comprised 13% of Canada's population in 2006, compared with 10% in 1981 and only 5% in 1921.

By 2056, the share of the population aged 65 and older may reach 27%.

Women were the majority among seniors—56% of persons aged 65 and older and 64% of those 80 and older in 2006.

Source: Statistics Canada – www.statscan.gc.ca

Chapter 1

Why Should Seniors Exercise?

When seniors engage in physical fitness every part of their body is included since it involves the workings of the heart, lungs, muscles, bones AND brain. Since what we do with our bodies also affects what we can do with our minds, fitness influences qualities of the entire being such as mental alertness and emotional stability. Before starting an exercise program it is always best to get your doctor's approval.

When we are involved in physical fitness it is like greasing the wheel, much like fine-tuning and good maintenance for a hard working engine. It enables us to perform to our full potential. Fitness can be most simply explained as a condition that helps us look, feel, and achieve our best out of daily living.

Being physically fit allows the body the ability to perform everyday tasks with energy and alertness. You also have enough vitality left over which allows you the capability for meeting urgent life circumstances, or enjoying hobbies and downtime activities. It provides the body with the power to go on, giving one the capability to cope with everyday life, especially having the power to withstand stress, to carry on in situations where an unhealthy person could not continue, and it is a major source for good health and well-being.

Studies show more and more that fitness levels clearly decline with age; a lot faster after age forty five. It is time to take charge of your senior years. Practicing this fitness driven behaviour can also improve the metabolic rate (the rate at which your body metabolizes the food you eat, or changes it into energy). The higher your metabolic rate, the more calories you burn at rest.

One of the reasons Americans and Canadians are living longer is because they are taking charge of their life. We are in better physical condition than our parents were at this age, primarily because physicians are constantly reminding today's senior citizens to be more aware of the need for exercise.

"Too often," says the ICAA, "people jump into exercise or try to do what they did 20 years ago, injuring themselves in the process. The 50-plus adult's physical capabilities and chronic diseases make this individual's needs different than those of a younger person." For this reason, I must reiterate the need to consult your doctor first and find a facility or trainer that will meet your personal needs. It is vital that you understand your limitations and obstacles as well as your potential.

Playing Active Video Games, (bodily interactive games) such as the Nintendo Wii games have shown to benefit seniors through moderate-intensity exercise. The investigative report is from the Sam and Rose Stein Institute for Research on Aging at the University of California, San Diego School of Medicine. In a pilot study, investigators found that use of exer-games substantially improved temper, frame of mind and mental health-related quality of life in older adults with SSD. (SSD is much more common than serious depression in seniors, and is connected with substantial anguish, functional disabilities, and increased use of costly medical services). Physical exercise can improve depression; however, fewer than five percent of older adults meet physical activity recommendations.

Exercise is THE best way to stimulate HGH (human growth hormone) in the body. HGH is a "youth" hormone that decreases as we age. Exercise stimulates the body to make lactic acid which in turn creates that hormone in the body.

More recent studies found that exercise helps cognitive skills (two studies), and it increases bone density in senior citizens (and non-seniors). People live longer, healthier, and happier lives if they exercise. Studies have shown that rheumatoid arthritis patients find power in exercise since it improves function, mental ability and alertness. It helps boost cognitive processing much faster, motor function and visual and auditory attention in healthy older people.

Studies using exercise to slow cognitive debility in older Americans find much success. Slowing Alzheimer's by one year could prevent 9.2 million cases, as the world prepares for 106 million victims by 2050. Aerobic exercise by older people helps to delay brain aging through better blood flow to the brain, as well as other organs. Routine exercise in senior citizens appears to prevent and improve mild cognitive impairment.

Walking as an exercise for older women provides positive results that can ease anxiety, stress and depression, because now she is breathing and moving.

Physical activity acts as a natural pain reliever for arthritis in Senior Citizens. Cardio-vascular exercise increases the flow of synovial fluid to the joints, helping to ease the pain of arthritis. This is great news for boomers since it can help them to stay off medications that can have serious side effects. Studies say it is possible to manage arthritis pain by moving more.

Osteoarthritis is caused by the wearing away of cartilage in the joints of the body, causing varying degrees of pain, stiffness and swelling. A greater number of Canadians will experience some sort of effect of this illness by age 70 while obese seniors may have a significantly higher lifetime risk. Many seniors with osteoarthritis find that Tai Chi exercise relieves pain, and helps them gain more fluidity in movement. Older runners are less likely to become disabled; they appear to survive longer.

Men who are active and are not afraid of work may have a decreased risk of prostate cancer. It is of upmost importance to remember that it is regular physical activity not occasional activity that is required to lower one's risk and to improve one's health. It is important that exercise becomes a lifestyle change.

Equally important to remember is the risk of colon cancer increases with age, nevertheless, with regular exercise routine and regular medical check-ups, it can be significantly reduced. Continuing to do the household chores and gardening among senior citizens are solutions that can meet some of their needs by helping them to keep their independence and mobility.

Older people who diet to lose weight without exercising, loose muscle mass needed for daily activities. As a rule, people tend to lose muscle mass as they become older but too much muscle loss will interfere with daily activities. Muscle mass in octogenarian women (women who are between eighty and ninety years of age) does not get stronger with exercise. In spite of this do keep in mind that exercise increases and improves spatial memory as well as the size of the brain structure in senior citizens.

German studies have revealed that physical activity has great anti-aging effects on the cardiovascular system. Cardio exercises could also be the answer to staying off medication permanently. Regular physical activity for older adults has been very effective in reducing heart disease, stroke, colorectal cancer, breast cancer and type two diabetes. Added benefits such as more daily exercise and fewer pounds in senior citizens may also reduce the risk of type II diabetes by half.

Physical activity is the foundation of any healthy lifestyle – especially for people with osteoarthritis. Exercise helps to maintain good joint health, manage their symptoms, and prevent the functional decline. Osteoarthritis, however, often makes physical activities, such as exercise, and performing daily activities, a challenge. "Activity strategy training" could offer patients with knee and hip osteoarthritis the chance to lead more active lives and steadily improve their overall health.

Being physically energized reduces stroke damage and speeds up the recovery process for Senior Citizens. The most energetic of these seniors –

average age 68 - also had a better chance of long-term recovery.

Chapter 2

Get the Green Light by Starting With A Checkup

With all these wonderful indications, you might want to JUMP right into exercise, but take caution. Think of how long it's been since you were active. Have you been active currently? What about recently? Can you recall the last time that you exercised? You must take your time in keeping with your own level of fitness.

Visit with your healthcare provider to find out whether you'll need to consider any special modifications to your exercise routine before starting a workout program. It is always a good idea to get an endorsement in order to begin a program. This can come in the form of a "PAR-Q" or Physical Activity Readiness Questionnaire. Most fitness facilities or trainers will have this form available for you, or you can download your own from this website:

www.csep.ca/english/view.asp?x=698

(Par-Q and You)

BMI Calculator

When you step onto the scale, the number it reads does not necessarily tell you your level of fitness or your true health. Body Mass Index (BMI) shows at a glance if extra pounds will translate into health risks, much like the Doctor Oz truth tube.

BMI indicates the relationship between weight and height. Higher numbers revealed on the scale equal a greater risk of developing health problems such as coronary artery disease, adult-onset diabetes and high blood pressure.

The metric formula for calculating your BMI is:
Your weight in Kilograms divided by (your height in meters squared)
For example: if you weigh 57 kg (about 126 lbs) and are 1.68 m tall (5'6") then:

57kg / (1.68 x 1.68) = BMI 20.21

BMI	Weight_Status
Below 18.5	Underweight
18.5 - 24.9	Normal
25 - 29.9	Overweight
30.0 & Above	Obese

Get acquainted with your options

There are many different strategies for beginning, and sticking to an exercise program. You need to know a few things about yourself first to get a better idea of where to begin. Before starting any program, investigate your alternatives and your strategy. What are your expectations from your fitness routine? Do you tend to be more alert and active in the morning or evening? Does indoor fitness appeal to you, or would you prefer to play outside? How much time will you dedicate to exercise? Make an honest list about the things that might keep you from being active and come up with a solution for each. Recognize that challenges can be overcome; you just need to be true to yourself above all else, plan to succeed.

Some individuals like to go to a gym and do a structured workout, while others enjoy a neighbourhood senior centre with group fitness classes. Ask yourself; is it more beneficial to spend money on joining a program? Alternatively, would you prefer to have a personal program developed by a trainer with whom you can do using objects or props in your home or office?   Many options are available.   Either option will help improve your fitness, and ability to function in life. Try to determine which method will meet your needs and goals.   There is no risk and your quality of life can greatly improve.   Be faithful and committed to regular exercise and with determination, you will achieve great results. Remember if you enjoy what you are doing, you will succeed at it, so find what you enjoy!

Thinking you'd like to work out with a group? Check out some facilities in your area. Visit your local YMCA or Seniors Centre, hospital-based fitness programs and city recreation programs or health club to view the types of offerings.   Visit facilities that offer cardio fitness and wellness programs.

When you visit the facility please take note of all the things that are important to you, and assess if they can meet your needs.   Does the facility feel friendly?   How private is the change room?   If the facility has a pool, what is the water temperature? About 84-88°F is comfortable for moderate to vigorous activity, while warmer temperatures can make exercise more difficult or potentially unsafe for some people.   Does the pool or workout room provide you with a safe way to enter and exit? Ask to try out some classes, so you can make a more informed decision about which program feels the most comfortable and fun while still giving you the workout you're looking for.

Observe the people who work in the facility and get a feel of how friendly they are, and whether they show any interest in you. Are they approachable and sociable, or are you just another "swipe-your-card" to them? Ask if the staff is qualified to work with older adults? Are all the instructors and personal trainers properly certified? Do they offer pre-exercise fitness assessments with periodic updates? Are they interested in helping you learn how to modify exercises to meet your fitness level and are they respectful of your needs? Do they encourage social interaction? Notice other mature adults in the facility and have a chat with someone who currently participates in the programs you're interested in. Get a feel for the general atmosphere.

Start Gently

Many people are eager to get started and can sometimes overdo it, which leads to pain, and can discourage them and set them up for failure. Appreciate that putting additional challenges on your muscles may lead you to be a little sore. Soreness should never last more than two days, and if it does, you should see your doctor immediately. Start slowly and avoid injuries. Work within your own abilities. Begin with light weights.

Figure out where in your day you will have time for fitness activities. Keep in mind those fitness activities aren't only performed indoors or with a trainer. Knowing how much time you can submit to fitness will help you in achieving your goal. Do this by recording all your activities during each

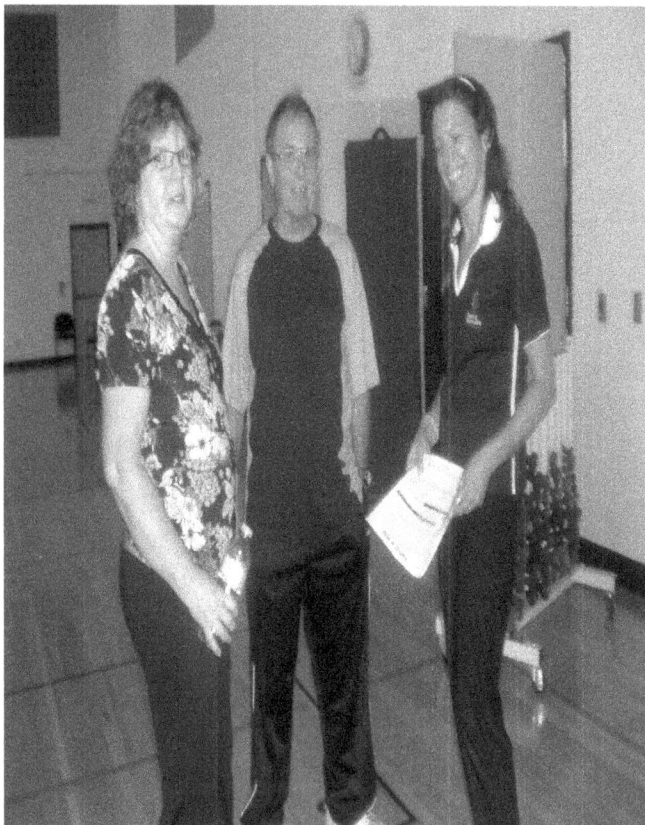

waking hour or for a day or two, tracking how much time you are sedentary (e.g. Sitting at your couch or desk) and active. (E.g. how much Walking you chose instead of driving to short errands). At the day's end, count how many hours you have not been physically active and look into scheduling some time slots for various activities that you could fit into your day.

Or you might wear a step counter throughout the day to count how many steps you take. This will give you a feel for how much you need to step up your game plan. Less active people tend to take about 4,000 steps or fewer per day. Aim to do 250 to 1,000 additional steps per day until you reach 8,000 to 10,000 steps in a day.

Alternatively, you might want to figure out your progress as you move through your fitness journey. Benchmark your progress by doing as many squats and pushups as you can. Record these numbers. Come back each month to squat and pushup again. Strive for improvement.

Chapter 3

Why Do YOU Want to Get More Fit?

Are you trying to lower your stress level or alleviate depression? Trying to maintain your independence? Maybe you're just making sure you can keep up with your grandchildren. Make a list and keep it in a highly visible place as a daily reminder of why you're doing this, along with a list of other long-term rewards. It will keep you motivated about attaining your long term goals. As you start to feel better physically you'll see yourself attaining these goals and that will increase your joy and laughter.

What kind of results should you expect from your physical activity program, and how does that correspond with your goals? Often people expect unrealistic results, such as losing loads of weight in a month. When these goals do not happen, many seniors may feel disappointed and relapse because they feel like they've failed. It will likely take more than a month to gain the weight so it will take more than a month to lose it. Remember anything worth doing will take a lot more effort than doing nothing at all. Fitness is not just about losing weight, it is about the numerous health benefits that come with being fit. Weight-loss is a by-product of exercise, but it isn't really the BEST thing that happens as your fitness level improves, it's just a bonus.

How Much Exercise Do I Need?

It is highly recommended for you to get clearance from your doctor before you begin any exercise program. Then it is advised that you seek the advice of a trained individual who will assess your level of fitness and help direct you to an appropriate program.

The Heart and Stroke Foundation says seniors, like most adults, need at least between 30 and 60 minutes of moderate activity most days of the week. Minutes count. Add up 30 or more minutes in 10 minute blocks. It is also important for seniors to do strength exercises for all their major muscle groups at least twice a week. This includes, but isn't exclusive to, chest and back, legs and butt, arms and abdominals. However, you must remember to allow your body to rest and recover and NEVER work the same muscle group 2 days in a row.

Start with light weights the first week, after which you can gradually increase your weight whenever necessary. It might be wise to start with small soup cans or no weights at all especially if you have not done any physical exercise for a long time. Starting with weights that are too heavy will cause injuries.

Over time, you can increase the amount of weight you lift in order to gain from these strength exercises. If you do not challenge your muscles, you will not increase your strength level and endurance. Challenge yourself to try to increase your weight in small increments, not more than 30% of the weight you currently lift. Furthermore, remember to allow your body to adapt to these higher levels of exercise slowly. Do not push yourself too hard. Work within your own body.

One "repetition" is one lift or push of a weight, apparatus or body part. One "set" equals 8 to 15 repetitions of an exercise. Adding an extra set is another way to increase your exercise intensity. Be mindful of your form and take your time lifting and lowering a weight. Avoid any jerky actions. When you move slowly, you work harder.

If it hurts, don't do it. Work around pain, not through it. Always breathe.

Many seniors are worried about getting enough exercise, especially since so much importance is being put on senior's fitness. However, it is possible to get too much exercise. Too much exercise may lead to over training, which can make you susceptible to injuries and illnesses. One of the things that can help you to stick to your workout plan is to understand the consequences before you ever come to them. This way you know what to look for and how to avoid falling off the "workout wagon".

Avoid multiple days a week of intense and difficult workouts. This can be hard on a body as repetitive motion leads to overuse injuries. It's always a better idea to mix it up a little, do some cross training. "Everything in moderation" is a great way to approach your training.

How Much Is Too Much?

When you began your exercise program you understood that everything takes time, and if it's worth doing, it's worth doing right. You've been working hard and really pushing yourself, but you're always tired and sore. You could be over training. If your workouts suddenly feel harder than usual, even though you haven't changed anything you could be over training. If you feel like you've hit a plateau or that your body has practically stopped responding to exercise all together, you might be over training. If you're feeling pain, it's time to re-assess your workout routine.

Symptoms of overtraining include;

- Insomnia

- Persistent muscle soreness

- Increased susceptibility to colds, sore throats and other illnesses

- Increased incidents of injuries – loss of coordination

- Loss of motivation or depression

- Elevated resting heart rate (morning pulse)

- Abnormal sweating

- Irritability / Indifference

- Loss in appetite

- Decrease in performance

If you come across any of these symptoms it's a good idea to discuss them with your physician to make sure that you are not overlooking something more serious that might be going on. If it is simply over training, what is causing it to occur and what can you do to avoid it?

The cause of over training is simple. You're not allowing your body adequate rest, and you might be repeating the same exercise too much! Your body needs time to recover and your muscle power will increase when you give your muscles enough time to rest and repair. Another cause might be that you are doing the same workout day after day which can also lead to over training, boredom and possible injury.

It is important to remember that when working with weights, do not work the same muscle group two days in a row. It is most important to remember to allow at least one day of rest before working the same muscle group again. You can do cardio exercise every day, but you should change your intensity with each workout. Jogging 5km, six days a week isn't easy on a body, but if you replace a couple of those jogs with an aquatic class (for instance), you'll be giving your body a deserved break, as well as working in a different way. Change your routine, if you are use to walking every day consider doing some swimming or cycling instead, on alternating days, and avoid the same routine every day. You'll stay motivated and won't be likely to become bored.

What about Water?

Water is your body's main chemical component and makes up about 60% of your body weight. Although no single formula fits all people, knowing why you need water will help you speculate how much water you need to drink every day.

Every system in your body needs water, for instance, it moistens the tissues in the eyes, mouth and nose. It regulates body temperature, lubricates joints, protects body organs and tissues, prevents constipation, flushes toxins out of vital organs, dissolves and carries nutrients to your cells.

If you are deficient in water then this can lead to dehydration, which can drain your energy. Signs and symptoms of dehydration include, but aren't limited to, thirst, dry mouth, loss of appetite, dark coloured urine, fatigue or weakness, chills, skin flushing, and dry skin.

If your deficiency in water is allowed to continue unabated, when the total fluid loss reaches 5% the following effects of dehydration are normally experienced:

- Increased heart rate
- Increased respiration
- Decreased sweating
- Decreased urination
- Increased body temperature
- Extreme fatigue
- Muscle cramps
- Headaches
- Nausea
- Tingling of the limbs

When the body reaches 10% fluid loss, emergency help is needed IMMEDIATELY! 10 percent fluid loss and above is often fatal! Symptoms of severe dehydration include:

- Muscle spasms
- Vomiting
- Racing pulse
- Shriveled skin
- Dim vision
- Painful urination
- Confusion
- Difficulty breathing
- Seizures
- Chest and Abdominal pain
- unconsciousness

Be very vigilant that these are not the only symptoms of severe dehydration that can occur, just the most common ones. Symptoms will differ from person to person because everybody is different.

Too often many people fail to drink enough water and eat enough food when they are engaged in workout programs. When you exercise, your body will need more water than it usually does. You must drink water to replace the fluid you lose from your body each day.

For instance, the average urine output for adults is about 1.5 liters (6.3 cups) a day. You lose close to an extra liter (about 4 cups) of water a day through breathing, sweating and bowel movements.

Food intake only accounts for 20 percent of your total fluid intake, so if you consume two liters of water or other beverages a day (a little more than 8 cups) along with your normal diet, you will typically replace your lost fluids.

Alternatively, you can try the "eight times 8" method. Drink eight 8oz glasses (about 1.9 lire) of water each day to replenish lost fluids.

Drinking too much water, however, can lead to a condition known as water intoxication, or to a related problem resulting from the dilution of electrolytes in the body, hyponatremia. (Hyponatremia is an electrolyte disturbance in which the sodium concentration in the serum is lower than normal).

When too much water enters the body, the tissues can swell with excess fluid.

Electrolytes which are your Sodium, Potassium chloride and water disproportion and tissue puffiness can cause your heart to be out of rhythm, may allow fluid to enter the lungs, and can cause fluttering eyelids. Swelling puts pressure on the brain and nerves, which can cause behaviors resembling alcohol intoxication. Enlargement of brain tissues can cause seizures, coma and eventually death, unless water intake is restricted and a hypertonic saline (salt) solution is administered. If treatment is given before the tissue swelling causes too much cellular damage, then a complete recovery can be expected within a few days.

It is important that you maintain a nutritious diet while completing an exercise program in order to attain the best possible results. Fuel up after exercise. Your body needs energy to recover and that comes from food. A combination of carbohydrates, protein and fat will give your body the energy it needs. Remember you cannot run your car without fuel.

Stretching your muscles after your workout is equally important. Tight muscles can often cause other muscles of your body to overcompensate, which can cause injury over time.

Take some time out, include into your timetable recovery days into your weekly routine. Listen to your body. If you're only a few minutes into your workout, and you're feeling tired and unmotivated or clock watching, go back home and rest or do a light yoga workout.

Finally remember to get enough sleep and allow your body to adjust.

Keep in mind the most beneficial thing you can do for yourself when you feel over training fatigue is to rest. It would be far more beneficial to your body to slow down and give yourself a week or so off from exercise and come back fresh and more focused than to continue over training and injure yourself! Without proper rest, the chance of stroke or other circulation problems increases. Most health experts' advice that one should exercise every other day or three times a week.

I should also mention that stopping excessive exercise suddenly can also create a change in your mood. Feelings of depression and agitation can occur due to withdrawal from the natural endorphins produced by exercise.

Physical exercise releases peptides, endorphins, and opiates that exhibit synergetic effects with other neurotransmitters, causing exercise euphoria, also known as "runners high", thus causing addiction to physical exercise and possibly decreased sex drive. Remember too much of one thing might be good for nothing.

Use the "KISS" Method: Keep It Super Simple

Try doing activities that recommend an assortment of endurance, strength-building and flexibility benefits, which are your best considerations.

- Endurance activities include walking, hiking, swimming, dancing, cycling and skating. These are very beneficial for your heart, lungs and circulatory system. Do your own household cleaning and yard chores? In a gym or workout facility, you might use the treadmill, elliptical trainer, rower, stepper, or join an aerobics class.

- Make your feet work for you. Make a special effort to park at the outer edges of the grocery store parking lot, rather than looking for the space closest to the door. Try walking up the first flight of stairs in a high-rise, rather than waiting for the elevator. Add another floor every week. Walk or cycle to the grocery store or other services when possible when the weather permits. Ride your bike to a neighbourhood friend's house. Carry the grandchildren when the opportunity presents itself. Every extra step counts and you can always walk in the malls in the winter. Keep your feet moving all the time.

- Participate in events, get involved, don't be one of the onlookers on the side lines. Once you're on your way to being better physically healthy, set a goal to participate in a charity event. Make plans to walk, run or bike to raise money for your favourite charity. Ask a friend to be your exercise and event partner. You will be elated just being with others that have the same goals in mind of taking charge of their wellness and well being.

- Flexibility activities can also be benefited from stretching, yoga, Tai Chi, raking leaves in the fall or even cleaning the lawn and vacuuming. They all keep your joints limber due to the increased flexibility which will keep you flexible enough to be able to continue to tie your shoes, reach the top shelf in your kitchen and clip your toenails.

- Reach for the top. Stretch for items from the highest shelf you can reach in the kitchen and closets and take the time to clean them. Do something that is out of the way or different chores each day that you might not have done without sacrificing your normal exercise routine. Do a little extra everyday tidy such as a shelf or reorganize your space.

- Stretch, walk, and march in place when doing dishes or any stationary jobs. Walk, stand and sit as many times as possible when you're talking on the phone or during TV commercials. Choose to do a hobby such as knitting, crocheting, and folding laundry, ironing or even doing puzzles when watching television to keep the mind and body active.

- Get involved in Strength activities, which simply include lifting light weights such as cans, climbing stairs, doing push ups against a wall in a standing position, or sitting down and standing up in rapid succession repeatedly. Any of these exercises will build weak muscles and improve balance and help in preventing falls, which is one of the leading causes of death from injury in people over 65. You're never too old to strengthen your body: Case studies have shown that weight training can reverse muscle weakness even among people in their 90s.

- Try focusing on all the major muscle groups in the legs, chest and back. Work out in such a way that you give special attention to your muscles and push them a little harder than they are accustomed to. However, you should do so in a gradual increase in a progressive manner. Understand that, like life, you only get out of exercise what you put into it, so exercise according to your desired expectations.

- Do balance exercises, as well as strength exercises? Which one should I choose or should I choose both? It is very important to have good balance to stop a mature senior from falling and suffering broken bones. Follow a well-rounded program possibly put together for you by a trained individual. Always warm up before performing exercises.

- Put in place a support network you can count on. Discuss your new goals with your friends and family and ask for their co-operation and encouragement. Involving others often helps us to keep our commitments. Put in place some telephone reminders from your support network to help keep you on track. Invite friends to work out with you while they visit such as walking around a few blocks.

- Reward yourself. Once you've accomplished your goal, treat yourself to something that reminds you of what a good job you've done and encourages you to continue, like going to see a good movie. Make it a reward that feeds your spirit such as watching a good comedy movie that can make you laugh a lot. However, you should not necessarily make an expensive purchase or food. Make more memories and laugh when you can.

Chapter 4

Group Exercise Classes for Fitness

IMPORTANT INFORMATION

Some instructors like to stop for pulse-checks. Others use the Perceived Exertion Chart (left), which asks you "on a scale of one to ten, how hard do you feel you are working?" Many industry professionals believe this is a better way because this scale is directly related to how you feel, not your heart rate. Some seniors take medications that help the heart maintain a steady rhythm, so the pulse check would not tell these individuals what they want to know. However, if you feel uncomfortable or dizzy, you will know right away and be able to respond accordingly.

Generally, any kind of fitness class should make you breathe heavier than normal, increases your heart rate (pulse), and make you feel warm or sweat. If you feel tired during the aerobics portion of the class, it is very important to keep your feet moving so that your blood doesn't pool in your feet. You can slow down your pace, lower your arms, or just march lightly until you feel a little better. If you need to sit and stop, tap your toes while you are seated. You should always work within YOUR abilities. You want to feel successful when you complete any kind of fitness activity so work at your own pace.

Group fitness classes are normally done to music that is between 108 and 150 beats per minute, depending on the activity. Slower music for slower classes like stepping or sculpting, a little faster for cardio or boot camp classes. Music plays a large part in fitness classes, as it is used to keep the class moving together, within the same rhythm much like a dance.

If you are a heart patient, or have had a cardiac event in the past, let your instructor know. If you have medication that you are required to carry with you, you should always let her or him know where you keep it. Then you should always keep it there. Please note this is nothing you should be embarrassed about. However, it is your instructor's business. She or he could save your life by having that little nugget of information.

Do's and Don'ts for Fitness Classes

- DO modify or slow down your movement when you are having difficulty maintaining proper form and posture. Ask the instructor for help when necessary.

- DON'T keep going if it hurts. Fitness shouldn't be painful or uncomfortable. Don't over think what you're doing, it's only movement.

- DO attempt to make arm movement as large and controlled as you can. Keep your chest up, shoulders down, and extend arms and legs fully.

- DON'T lock your knees or round your shoulders. Keep a tall, athletic posture in all your movements.

- DO keep your head in line with your spine, and keep your spine long.

- DON'T crane your neck or look up toward the ceiling as this puts undue stress on the cervical spine. Keep your head aligned with your spine.

The only time you should look at the ceiling is when you're lying on your back.

- DO keep heels, shins and knees aligned at all times, and keep all toes on the floor when supporting weight. Furthermore, make sure that your knees and feet face the direction that your body is facing.

- DON'T let your knees go past your toes when performing squats or lunges, as this will put undue stress on your knees. Keep knees directly over heels.

- DO hold abdominal muscles firmly throughout the class for proper posture and back-support.

- DON'T slouch or sway your back. Pull belly-button through toward your spine, and shoulders down toward your "back pockets".

- DO move slowly and in control. Keep wrists aligned with the forearm. Keep the upper body (neck & shoulders) relaxed throughout the exercise.

- DON'T let the weight you are using pull your hands out of alignment. Keep the back of your wrist flat not folded back. You are in control of the weights in your hands, not the other way around. Furthermore, don't squeeze the weight tightly as this engages the forearm muscles unnecessarily.

- DO think about and maintain body alignment from head to toe. Exercise should not feel awkward. All movements are natural and smooth.

- DON'T work beyond your own limitations. Be in YOUR body and work with what you have.

- DO smile and enjoy yourself.

- DON'T compete with anyone in the class.

If your hearing isn't so good, move closer to the instructor. If you have impaired vision you should move right to the front of a class. Sometimes following the person in front of you ISN'T the next best thing to do. Make sure you can see and hear the instructor. After a few weeks, when you're used to her/his teaching style you can move to wherever you like because you'll know a little better what to look forward to.

Be sure that your expectations are realistic. It is very possible you might not be able to keep up with the rest of the class at first, but don't let that discourage you. Even the most elite athletes have to walk before running.

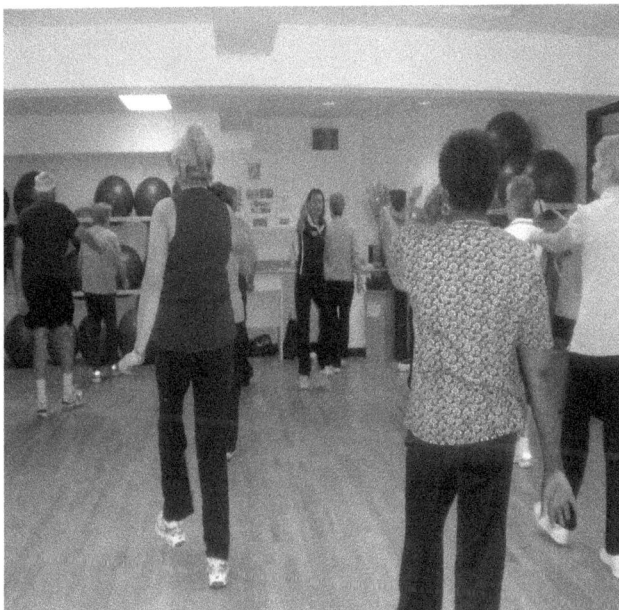

There are so many different styles and classifications of group fitness classes, how will you know which one is right for you? Following is a brief description of many types of classes, and what you might expect from each kind. Ultimately though, you will want a class or activity that you will enjoy, either from a physical or social sense. Sometimes just going to a class because your best friend goes is good enough. Just get out there and move.

Walking, Nordic Walking, Pole Walking

If you enjoy walking, you can turn an unhurried stroll into as much exercise as you'd like. It's a healthy way to increase your overall fitness, health and wellness - and people at all fitness levels can do it and it's FREE! No costly equipment is necessary, just a pair of shoes (and feet, of course) and you're on your way! Like all other exercises, using the proper form ensures maximum benefits and reduces your chance of exercise-related injuries.

Walking can help you improve your overall fitness and health, improve your mood, keep your bones and muscles strong, decrease your risk of heart attack and stroke, keep your blood pressure in check and help control your weight. Why not walk?

Nordic walking, or 'poling', uses two specially designed poles that work the upper body while walking. Poles are used to match each step you take, thereby engaging the arm, chest and upper back muscles through a full range of motion, stretching muscles that are often tight. The 'opposite arm to opposite leg' movement with poles engages abdominal/back muscles. Poling increases your heart rate without increasing your perceived exertion. Your heart rate increases much the same as it would by walking faster, however some people do not want to walk faster or cannot walk fast.

Before you start, get fitted with the proper shoes. The appropriate shoe, with the suitable fit, will help you to get the most out of your walking experience and save you later aches and pains.

How to Walk:

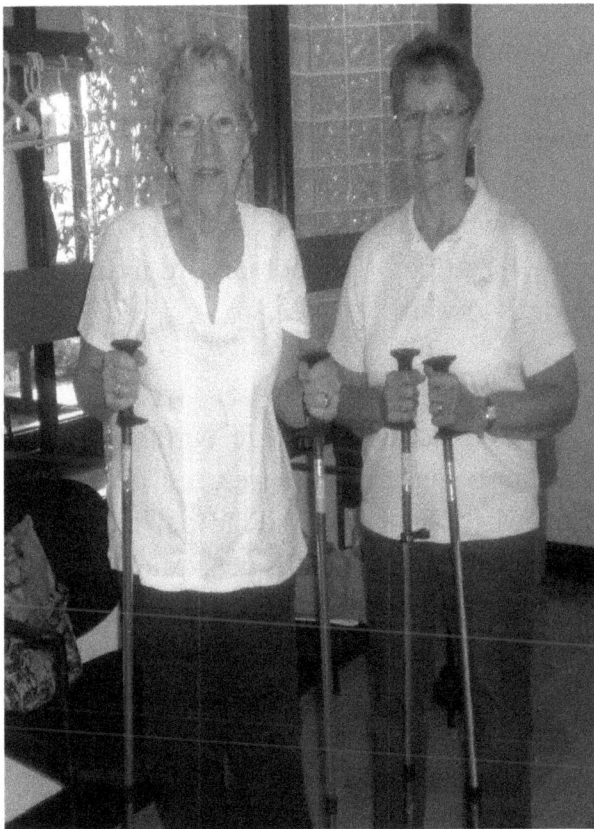

With your initial step, your heel should make first contact with the ground. Roll your foot forward in a smooth motion. Your toes are the last part of your foot to touch the ground and subsequently the last part of your foot to leave the ground as you move forward. Push off with your toes to give you forward momentum.

Swing your arms. Bend your elbows to 90-degrees. Keep your hands relaxed. Keep your shoulders relaxed. Keep your elbows close to your body. Swing your arms in a forward and back motion. Swing your arms in an 'opposite arm to opposite leg' stride. Left foot forward means right arm swings forward.

Where to Pole:

Fitness grade Nordic poles are portable, in that they collapse inside themselves. They can be used anywhere you walk. Find out if your city has some bike/walking paths near your home and discover their distance. Then go for a walk. Maybe you're planning a trip to the zoo with the grandkids, or any local attraction. In the colder months, take your poles with you to a mall or marketplace, just to walk around (although I don't recommend this during the holiday season when the malls are full of shoppers).

People may wonder why you have ski poles in your hands, but they're the ones who haven't heard about this fast growing fitness trend. You might be surprised at how many other people you meet with poles in their hands while you're out walking.

Be sure to stretch your upper and lower legs about 10 minutes into your walk, and again at the end of your walk. This will help keep your muscles supple and flexible, avoiding cramps and tightness.

Chair-ercise, Chair-Fit, Sit-Fit

Just because you're not as mobile as you used to be doesn't mean you should stop exercising all together. Seated exercise is designed to keep you moving! Move your legs and arms while seated to increase your heart rate, improve your range of motion, condition your muscles, and have a little fun.

Equipment used in this class consists of an armless chair, (arms on chairs can get in the way and limit your movement), resistance tubing or dyna-bands, light weights, play balls, small squeeze balls, light body bars, or any kind of light resistance such as soup cans or paper plates.

The goal is to increase your heart rate using simple functional movement, and light resistance moves to challenge strength and endurance.

This class generally begins with some seated marching or walking to music, with arms moving, then continues with some light muscle conditioning/resistance training in order to help strengthen muscles and increase range-of-motion (joint flexibility is defined as the range of motion - ROM - allowed at a joint). There may also be some standing exercises, depending on the overall mobility of the participants. This is a functional training class, in that it is designed with exercises which train the body for everyday activities.

You might feel warm or even sweat in this class. Use the perceived exertion chart as an indicator of how hard you are working. If you feel like you are working too hard, just slow down your pace, keep your feet moving lightly or toes tapping. Keep this pace till you feel better, then join in with the class again when you are able.

Chapter 5

What is Osteofit?

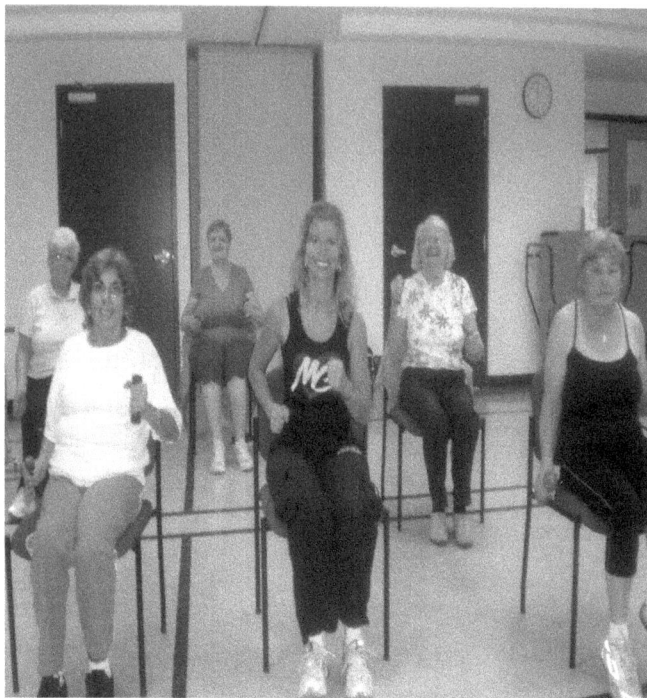

Osteofit is intended to improve strength, balance and coordination as well as increase your ability to cope with daily activities, independence, and quality of life. It is especially safe for those with osteoporosis, osteoarthritis, Osteopenia, Ankylosing spondylitis and other conditions that affect joints and bones.

Osteoporosis is a condition in which abnormal loss of bony tissue resulting in frail porous bones is brought on by a lack of calcium. It is very common in postmenopausal. This disease of the bone leads to an increased risk of fractures. It affects one in four women and one in eight men over 50, according to the osteofit website.

Osteopenia is the name given to bone mineral density (BMD) that is lower than normal peak BMD but not low enough to be classified as osteoporosis.

Ankylosing spondylitis (AS) is an ever present inflammatory form of arthritis that affects the spinal joints. The characteristic feature of AS is the connection of the joints at the base of the spine where the spine joins the pelvis - the sacroiliac (SI) joints.

The disease course is highly inconsistent, and while some individuals have episodes of transient back pain only, others have more chronic severe back pain that leads to differing degrees of spinal stiffness over time. In most cases, the disease is portrayed by acute painful episodes and remissions (periods where the problem settles).

Osteofit should be attended twice per week for a minimum of 6 weeks. This registered program of one-hour classes includes an educational component with topics on fracture prevention and healthy living. The exercise programme focuses on improving strength, posture, balance and agility, through the use of practical exercises, agility activities, resistance training and appropriate stretches.

Find weekly or bi-weekly, hour-long registered or drop-in sessions, consisting of a 15-minute warm-up, exercises with resistance bands and weights, squats and lunges, balancing exercises and rubber ball games designed to improve co-ordination and agility. The exercises are made up of a combination of yoga, tai-chi, mat Pilates, and strength training, core stability, and balance. No dangerous gyrations or high-impact moves are used. Relaxation techniques will include visualization, breathing exercises, and contract-relax techniques. The program is designed to simply be fun and safe exercises are choreographed to music.

Your instructor will be able to teach and define the condition of osteoporosis and its harmful effects on self reliance and quality of life, as well as;

- Review classifications of osteoporosis.

- Review the economic burden of this disease condition on society.

- Recognize risk factors for osteoporosis.

- Pinpoint the treatment options for the management of osteoporosis.

- Identify lifestyle behaviors that can be modified to decrease the risk of falls.

- Explain the role of exercise in decreasing the incidence of falls.

- Explain age related physiological changes among older adults.

The osteofit instructor will show and demonstrate safety in all aspects of preparation and method of the Osteofit program, as well as demonstrate a technique for avoiding and managing injuries.

- For a given exercise, analyze its intended purpose, potential risks to joint structures, and provide modifications or alternative exercises.

- Describe and demonstrate correct body alignment.
- Demonstrate the principle of exercise progression for a given muscle group.
- Implement the principle of specificity to effectively select the appropriate exercise option for the participant's level of ability.
- Identify exercises, which have the potential to cause injury.
- Identify activities with a high risk for falling.
- Describe the responsibilities and legal liabilities of the instructor/facility associated with the participant's personal injury and specific medical background, and physical activity screening methods (i.e. Pre-screening methods such as the Par-Q).
- Give precautionary measures for beginning exercise participants that are designed to prevent injury and increase safety for all components of fitness.
- Know the set of emergency procedures for the facility and the employer such as first aid, support procedures, medical referral procedures, and follow up.
- Describe the Osteofit instructor's professional limitations regarding the physical activity

participation of adults who are not apparently healthy.

- Describe the Osteofit instructor's professional limitations for providing information on medical conditions and nutrition.

What are the benefits of these Classes?

You will work to strengthen bones to prevent disease, and reduce bone fractures.

Your instructor will define powerful muscles and how to burn more calories and improve physical health, lose weight or maintain weight, how to work towards a healthy heart and how you can reduce the risk of heart disease, reduce blood pressure, boost immune system and improve blood circulation.

You will be taught the importance of good posture in order to prevent injuries and have a healthy back, core strength and pelvic floor muscles. You will be taught stretches, yoga and Pilates exercises, all of which will be incorporated in the class.

You will be able to improve co-ordination and balance to enhance motor skills by improving balance and learning 'moves' to music.   You will benefit from brain exercise from learning simple dance type 'routines' that are fun but easy.   Like all fitness classes, it improves all levels of fitness, depending on your intensity.   Osteofit exercise can be as easy or as hard as you want to make it.

It teaches you exercises you can do anywhere without the use of machines and equipment, i.e. how to adopt the exercise as part of your lifestyle for quality, well being and longevity.

Social interaction – You will be able to meet a new set of friends.   Some participants will have been doing the class for several years and will be very friendly and welcoming.   They are a celebration of above average bone density for their age group. They will encourage you along and new bonds of friendship will be formed.

Low Impact - Easy-Fit – Light Aerobics – Beginner Fitness

One foot is always on the ground in this type of class, meaning no jumping or jarring movements. Classes like these are great for beginners because they are generally of a lower intensity and made up of easier movements and exercises.   It's also a great way to ease into fitness, or get back into exercise after some time away from it. Comprised of a warm-up, aerobic component, cool down and stretch, and can include a resistance training component, these classes are designed to burn calories, increase cardio-vascular health, and improve muscle strength and endurance with as little impact to the joints as possible.

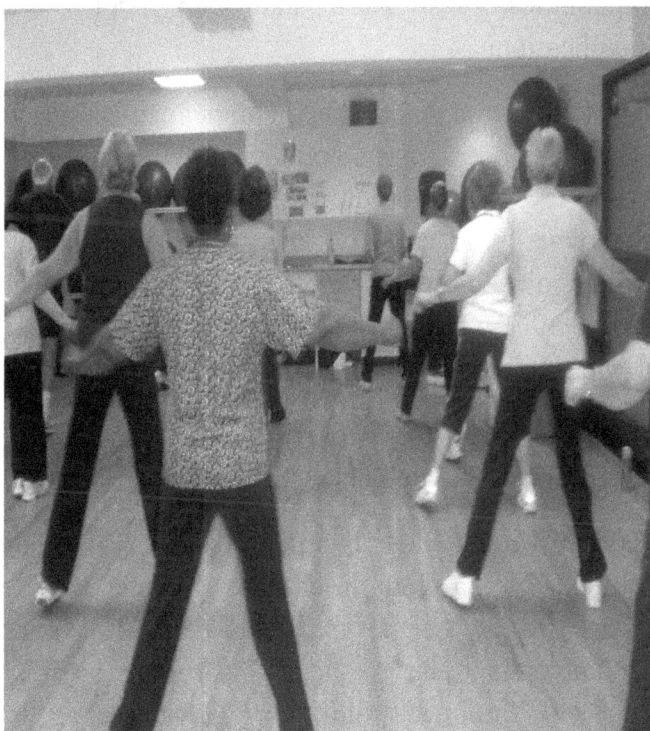

This class will increase your core temperature and make you sweat. Your heart rate will go up and you will breathe heavier. A little co-ordination helps but shouldn't be necessary for this class containing knee raises and hamstring curls, grapevines and heel-jacks. Arm movements in this class should be big and as full as you can make them, however never work beyond your own capabilities. Your instructor will offer modifications.

If you feel uncomfortable, light headed or dizzy, slow down but do not stop moving. A light march and a few deep breaths might help, if not take a seat where you can and keep your toes tapping while you sit comfortably, breathing normally. Drink some water. The instructor will assist you if you need help. Join back with the class when you feel you can.

Step Class – Riser Class – Stair-robics

Basically a step class is an aerobics workout that happens with a platform or step. The step can be from 4"to 20" high, your choice. The riser actually has built in shock absorption, so it is easier on the knees than you might expect. In addition to stepping up and down on the step, participants are expected to move their arms and incorporate other moves that work the whole body.

This class will make you sweat as you use the bigger muscles in the thighs to lift yourself up on to, and lower yourself off of the step. Although each step class is unique to the instructor, they all start with the same basic moves. Beginner step classes will show you the very basics of step aerobics including how to step on the step, the music speed, what to do if you need a break. Don't let choreography scare you away. If you keep it up you'll be a pro in no time!!

The recommended music speed for stepping is between 120-128 beats per minute (bpm) or less. It becomes less safe to step with music faster than 128 bpm. Some people think they will get a better workout by going faster, but in reality for stepping, the slower, the better. Don't be tempted by speed. With speed comes momentum, and momentum isn't always your friend. It also isn't recommended to do step classes more than 4 times a week as it is a strenuous activity. 2 or 3 times a week is plenty.

Because this class uses such big muscles, it is demanding a LOT of oxygen so your heart is working hard. Think of the perceived exertion chart, and your oxygen debt. Are you feeling good or do you need to slow down? It is so important to keep your feet moving, especially in a class that is really working your heart. As with any fitness class, if you feel dizzy or distressed, let someone know right away. If you need to sit and drink water, keep tapping your toes or lifting your knees up while you sit to try to ease your heart rate back to a comfortable level

Dancercise – Dance Aerobics – Zumba

You don't have to be a disco queen or a hard-core clubber to succeed at dance style aerobics. These classes are essentially a mix of aerobics with dance moves and designed to increase heart rate, range of motion, strength and endurance.

Most cardio dance is based on a few simple steps which can be easily learned in the social atmosphere of a class. You don't have to have a highly developed sense of rhythm or a background in ballet. Just an ability to count and an openness to having a good time while getting fit. After all, it's just dancing! Your feet move, your arms move, but no-one expects you to be Baryshnikov. If your arms and legs simply refuse to work together, then keep your arms down and focus on what your legs are doing. When your feet know what to do, you'll be able to add the arms.

The Zumba® program fuses rhythmic Latin beats and easy-to-follow moves to create a fun and exciting fitness class. The routines include gaps of training sessions where fast and slow rhythms and resistance training come together to tone and sculpt your body while burning fat. Add some Latin sounds and international enthusiasm into the mix and you've got a Zumba® class!

In the past years, the Zumba craze has become quite a revolution, spreading like wildfire, and placing itself as the single most infectious movement in the industry of fitness.

As with any class, your heart rate will increase as well as body temperature. Take your time and ease into your first few classes but if you do feel overwhelmed, lightheaded or dizzy, slow down, keeping your feet moving lightly. Sit if you need

to and tap your toes. Join back with the class
when you feel better.

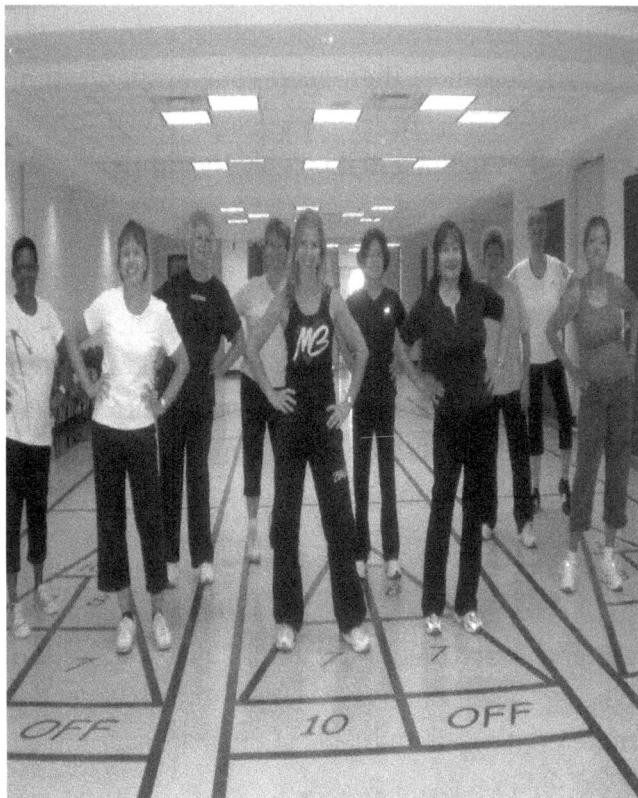

These cardio classes are designed to burn calories, increase range of motion and endurance, stimulate brain cells and be fun!

Spinning – Cycle-Fit

Spinning is an aerobic exercise that is done on a specially designed stationary bicycle called (obviously enough) a spinning bike. As you pedal, motivating music plays and your instructor takes you on a visualization of an outdoor cycling workout, (for example, "You're going up a long hill now, you can't see the top yet." etc). During the class you are constantly adjusting your pace -- sometimes motoring as fast as you can in "low gear", other times cranking up the tension and pedaling slowly from a standing position. This helps you to focus inward and work on your mind as well as your body.

The average spinning exercise class lasts 45 minutes, making use of varying speeds and resistance levels to provide a great cardiovascular challenge. Varying speed and intensity by changing resistance levels makes spinning an ideal way to develop and improve cardiovascular fitness. Regular participation in spinning classes increases the efficiency of the heart and lungs, improving blood flow and increasing oxygen distribution throughout the body. This is a fun but also a significant way to get fit and build up your leg muscles.

Although you can adjust your spin cycle to suit your fitness level, this is not really a form of exercise for the faint hearted. The emphasis in this class is to push yourself harder and faster to build up your overall fitness. It is very beneficial for your heart and lungs as well as your growing endurance level and overall strength in your body; however it is a high intensity class.

Know that you are in control of your intensity. These classes can be very challenging, especially for beginners. Using the bigger muscles of the body puts a high demand on the heart. Take the time to start slowly and easily, and then work your way up at your own pace. Remember, even champions had to start slowly in their sport.

If you need to take a break, slow down or get off the bike and walk around till you feel better. Join in with the class when you feel you can.

Boot Camp – Extreme Fitness

The phrase "Boot Camp" usually indicates a very high intensity class; however you can control the intensity at which you work. Just because the instructor is jumping up and down doesn't mean you must also do so. However the premise behind the boot camp is that you push yourself hard and to your limits to get your body in shape through discipline and dedication. It's a positive and healthy way to burn up energy, and can be enjoyed and endured by old and young people alike.

The boot camp doesn't mean you'll become a soldier by the end of the session, but that you will work hard with focus and energy that will kick start a whole new attitude to a healthier and fitter lifestyle. It's about setting and meeting challenges that are highly satisfying to achieve.

This class focuses on keeping your heart rate elevated in order to burn more calories and improve your intensity. The exercises are demanding and concentrate on working your cardiovascular system intensely. Workouts include jumping jacks, burpees, running up hills or stairs and other body weight callisthenic exercises. The idea is to burn a lot of calories as capably as possible. The best way to do that is to move hard!

Again be aware of how hard you are working and if you need to lower your intensity, do so. Don't come to a complete stop just make smaller easier movements until you feel better.

Sculpting – Body Shaping – Weight Training

If you want to get in shape, weight training or sculpting needs to be part of your fitness program. True conditioning includes a combination of cardio, strength and flexibility training, all of which are equally important to your overall health and well being.

Any class listed as a "Sculpt" or "Tone" class is going to be made up of resistance exercise that will challenge your muscle strength and endurance. It is an anaerobic class designed to build muscle. This class usually begins with a warm up of 5-15 minutes then continues with exercises that challenge all the major muscle groups in the body, as well as some functional weight training exercise.

people think about weight training, they
liately equate it to bodybuilding, and many
: are afraid to include weights in their
ım for fear they'll bulk up.   Understand that
uilders spend about 8 hours every day
ıg to get bigger.   It's their job to get big.
ob in the gym is just to increase the amount
ı muscle mass on your body.

nuscle burns more calories at rest than fat.
ng more muscle mass on your body raises
 metabolism, increasing the number of
:s your body burns at rest.   There's even
evidence that increasing muscle mass will
se bone mass.

 researchers at McMaster University in
ton, Ontario studied a group of
enopausal women on a year-long program of
ɔbic strength training, not only did their
e size increase by 20 percent, but their
 bone mass rose by 9 percent. It's possible,
that strength training might help defend
:t   osteoporosis.
alnews.com/010528.html)

Martial Arts

Tai Chi-Tae Bo - Fitness Boxing – Kickboxing – Combat Fitness

You don't have to be Bruce Lee to reap martial arts benefits. A blanket term that covers many disciplines like judo, jujitsu, tae kwon do, karate, ninjitsu, kung fu and tai chi, martial arts started out as forms of unarmed combat used mainly in Asia.

The aim is not only to get fit but also to ensure that the body and mind are spiritually in tune. It's about discipline and respect as well as knowing the moves themselves. Many practitioners train for years working their way up through different levels that are sometimes represented by wearing different coloured belts.

Martial arts is not just fitness, it really is a way of life and demands deep commitment and dedication. However, now there exist classes that take many of the moves from these martial arts disciplines, which have been simplified and set to music.

These classes tend to be high intensity cardiovascular endurance challenges which means you will breathe heavily and your heart rate will go up. As with all classes, be aware of how hard you are working and if you need to lower your intensity, do so. Don't come to a complete stop just make smaller easier movements until you feel better.

With a range of kicking and punching together with intermittent speed drills, you will work hard. A class made up of punching and kicking is a great way to work out frustrations while you burn lots of calories.

Always be sure to keep elbows and knees, "soft" when punching and kicking. That means your joint is NEVER straight, there is always a slight bend to it. Even when you push your arm out fully to throw a jab, your elbow never comes out straight.

A fist is made by closing the thumb around the fingers, not the other way around, and punches tend to be palm-down. Kicks 'lead' through the heel, meaning you don't flick your leg and point the toe. Foot is flexed and pushed out and in from a bent knee position.

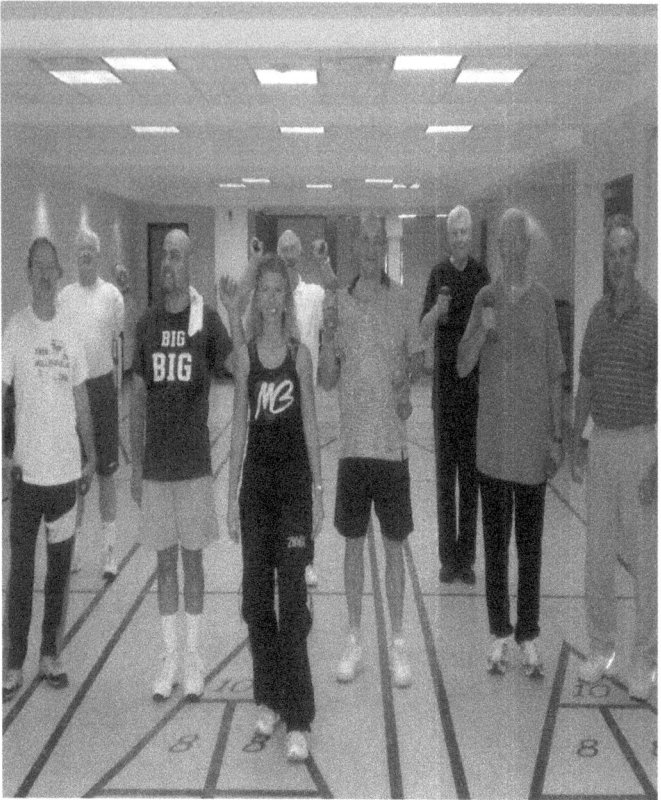

Chapter 6

What is Tai Chi?

Tai chi is an ancient Chinese martial art involving a series of slow, controlled and meditative body movements that were originally designed for self-defense and to promote inner peace and calm. Tai chi is a centuries-old Chinese martial art that came down from qigong, an ancient Chinese discipline that has its roots in traditional Chinese's medicine. If you are ever in China take a stroll to the park and you will see people that are moving gracefully; they are practicing this art.

Tai chi has been shown to help develop balance, strength, endurance, aerobic capacity, and self-confidence and prevent falls in seniors. It has also been found that it reduces fibromyalgia symptoms and reduces stress.

In traditional Chinese's medicine, human beings are considered miniature versions of the universe, and like the universe, they are thought to be made up of the constant interaction of five elements. These elements are metal, water, fire, wood, and earth. It is believed that these five elements flow in a unified manner throughout all the organs of the body as the five phases of universal Qi (pronounced "chee"), with qi represented as the life force—the natural energy in the body that travels along channels in the body called meridians. Health is achieved when the exchanges between these elements cause the flow of your qi to occur in a smooth and balanced manner. You could say that one motivation for people studying tai chi is to help your qi flow effortlessly.

Yang, wu, and tai chi chih are three of the most common styles of tai chi. The yang style includes 108 movements in the traditional form and 24 movements in its simple form. Please note that it is demanding because you must keep your stance wide and your knees bent most of the time; the wu style, which includes 100 movements in the traditional style and 24 to 36 movements in its shorter form. It is gentler because it uses a narrow, elevated stance where the knees are not bent as much as the yang style; and the tai chi chih style, which has 20 movements, also uses a more elevated stance, but with much less transfer of weight from one leg to the other than the other two.

Tai Chi, as it is practiced in the west today, has often been thought of as a moving form of yoga and meditation combined. It is a combination of a sequence of movements; many of these movements are originally derived from the martial arts. Martial art tai chi is mainly about —slow, musical, contemplative actions intended to help you find peace and calm. For the participant, the focus in doing them is not, first, martial, but as a meditative exercise for the body. The aims of Tai Chi are to promote the circulation of this 'chi' within the body, the belief since by doing so the health and vitality of the person are improved.

One of the main purposes of Tai Chi is to cultivate a calm and tranquil mind, focused on the precise performance of these exercises. Learning to practice Tai chi benefits such things as balance, alignment, fine-scale motor control, rhythm of movement as well as the origin of movement from the body's vital center. The participant learns the importance of aligning the body.

The practicing of Tai Chi may very well to some degree contribute to being able to stand longer and more upright, (walk, move, run, etc.) in other areas of life as well. People who practice Tai Chi become more conscious in terms of correcting poor postural, alignment or movement patterns, which can contribute to tension or injury. In addition, the contemplative nature of the exercises is calming and relaxing, in and of itself.

Since the Tai Chi movements have their beginnings in the martial arts, practicing them does have some martial applications. In a two-person exercise known as 'push-hands' Tai Chi's main beliefs are developed in terms of being receptive to and reactive to another person's 'chi' or central energy. It is also a chance to employ some of the martial aspects of Tai Chi in a kind of slow-tempo combat. The importance in Tai Chi is on being able to channel potentially destructive energy (in the form of a kick or a punch) away from one in a manner that will scatter the energy or send it in a direction where it is no longer a danger.

Some participant claims that it is believed that tai chi can delay aging and prolong life, increase flexibility and strengthen muscles and tendons, and aid in the treatment of heart disease, high blood pressure, arthritis, digestive disorders, skin diseases, depression, cancer, and many other illnesses. Unfortunately, there hasn't been a great deal of scientific evidence to support all of these claims.

Because tai chi actions are slow and purposeful with shifts of body weight from one leg to the other in harmonization with upper body movements (sometimes with one leg in the air), it challenges balance and one could imagine that it would help improve balance and reduce falling incidence in seniors.

It was noted that individuals who practiced tai chi walked significantly more steps than individuals who did not. Walking is clearly linked with a decreased risk of cardiovascular disease, diabetes, and other chronic illness, and so if tai chi can improve walking, then it's certainly worth giving it a try.

Here are some reasons to practice Tai Chi

- Movements are low-impact and gentle and put minimal stress on your muscles and joints.
- The risk of injury is very low.
- You can do it anywhere, anytime.

- It requires very little space (no excuses apartment dwellers!) and no special clothing or equipment.
- You do it at your own pace.
- It's noncompetitive.
- It can be done in groups or by yourself
- There are lots of movements to keep you interested, and as you become more accomplished you can add those to your routine.

You should wear comfortable and loose-fitting clothing that won't restrict your movements. Sweat pants, tights, or leotards, and a T-shirt will do work just fine. Although to the untrained eye it doesn't look like lots of work, because the movements are so deliberate, you may work up a sweat, and so it is best not to overdress.

That is Tai Chi. Practicing this exercise frequently can enhance your aerobic capacity, muscular strength, flexibility, and balance; and it can improve your well-being and decrease your stress. It's a martial art that has been around for centuries and is followed by millions of Chinese. If this style appeals to you, at least try it, you just might benefit from it. Yoga – Pilates – Nia are all mind and body exercises.

Chapter 7
What is Yoga?

YOGA – The Path to Union, the word yoga means "union" in Sanskrit. What is commonly referred to as "Yoga" can be more correctly described by the Sanskrit word "Asana", which refers to the practice of physical postures or positions. Yoga is

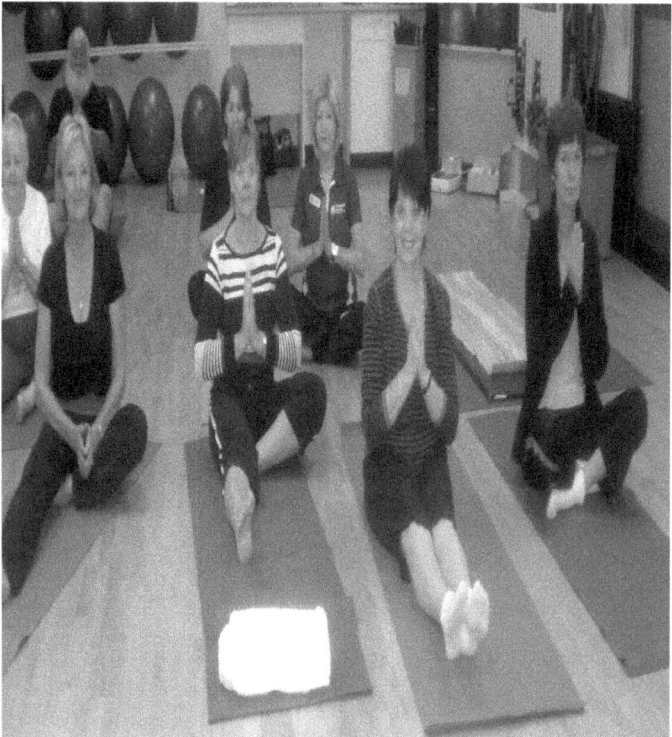

a systematic science; its teachings are an integral part of good health and wellbeing. Yoga teaches one not to DO but to BE.

Yoga has evolved over 5000 years and is now being embraced globally because of its many benefits. It is a gentle approach to an ANCIENT ART, designed to work with the body you have today.

It is a harmonious relationship of BODY, MIND, BREATH, and SPIRIT which is the foundation for GOOD HEALTH. By combining specifics postures called ASANAS, deep breathing called PRANAYAMA and relaxation techniques called SAVASANA, we create a balance of body, mind and spirit.

Yoga will bring you energy and vitality. It cleanses by releasing the body toxins. Most of all it will help you to still and calm a busy mind opening you to new and creative ideas. Yoga will strengthen the nervous and endocrine systems. In addition, your muscles and joints will become stronger and more flexible. Regular practice of yoga will benefit lower back pain, arthritis, osteoporosis, high blood pressure, menopause, PMS, pregnancy and many other ailments.

For senior citizens one of the better ways to stay fit and healthy is by practicing some Yoga exercises. Make sure you choose a yoga instructor that you're comfortable with and who meets your needs. There is no harm in checking out different instructors. Remember you are the one paying the fee so make sure you are going to get what you want out of the program. Each instructor will have his or her own way of leading their class through the postures, but you might want to choose a very gentle and patient person who is used to working with seniors.

If you have made a decision to practice yoga here are some helpful tips:
- Wear loose clothing
- Exercise on an empty stomach
- Aim to practice regularly
- Practice your breathing and relaxation
- Take your time and make your movements slow and fluid

Benefits of Regular Yoga Practice

When Yoga is practiced regularly, it helps decrease the negative burden of stress on the mind and body. It can most definitely aid the body in coping with age. Growing old is also the time when you are more susceptible to some aches and pains. Yoga can do a lot to help ease some of this discomfort.

Increasing Flexibility – yoga has various positions that have a direct effect upon the various joints of the body including those joints that are never really in your thoughts until they start to pain you. Yoga helps in increasing lubrication of the joints, ligaments and tendons while the yoga positions exercise the different tendons and ligaments of the body.

Massaging of the Organs of the Body – Yoga is possibly the only form of exercise which can effectively massage all the internal glands and organs of the body in a thorough manner of which include the prostate. In reality, the prostate hardly receives any external stimulation during one's entire lifetime! Yoga is a healthy approach of stimulation on the various body parts. This stimulation and massage of the organs has its payback by warding off disease and providing a forewarning at the first possible sign of a likely beginning of a disease or a disorder.

Complete Detoxification –Ss is a result of gently stretching muscles and joints as well as massaging the various organs. Yoga makes certain that the optimum supply of blood reaches the various parts of the body. This helps in flushing out toxins from every hidden corner of the body as well as providing nourishment to these areas. This has a tremendous benefit on our health because it helps in delaying age. It can surely provide an abundance of energy and an incredible zest for life.

Toning of the Muscles – Muscles that happen to be saggy, weak or flabby are stimulated repeatedly while toning to shed excess weight and droopiness.

Your yoga class might start with a short time of relaxation either sitting or lying down. There may be relaxing music in the background. Bear in mind that your teacher is aware that you are new to these exercises. They will reinforce you to "listen to your body".

You will be asked to breathe gently and deeply. Then your coach or teacher will walk you through relaxation exercises, releasing the spine to the ground, softening the face, concentrating on your breath and your body and how you are feeling, acknowledge the aches and pain and let it go, filling your senses with the music. You should start to release, relax and let go. This will last anywhere from five to fifteen minutes. This is called Savasana.

Next there will likely be some gentle warm up exercises such as circling the wrist, ankle and gently moving the head from side to side. Then you may be asked to take the knees into the chest rocking from side to side, perhaps to take your limbs up in the air and make wide circles in both directions, but doing only what your body will let you do that day, knowing that your teacher or coach will have modified poses for those who need it.

Then you'll gently move on to some flexibility exercises, such a soles of the feet together with knees bent and arms out in "T" with the spine released to the ground and you are breathing gently. You will feel your hips opening up and your upper back will start to loosen. In your chest, your heart will start to lift and lighter. When you keep your breath soft, your throat and jaws will also soften. You will experience a sense of peace in your inner core.

You will then slowly and gently move through a series of asanas, or postures. During this time, your instructor will talk you through and show your modifications if necessary. The idea is to have one pose flow gently into the next pose without any jerky motions. The challenge is in the slowness and fluidity of the movement.

You will also be led through a series of stretches that are designed to lengthen your spine and focus on breathing. Your session will end with breathing and stretching.

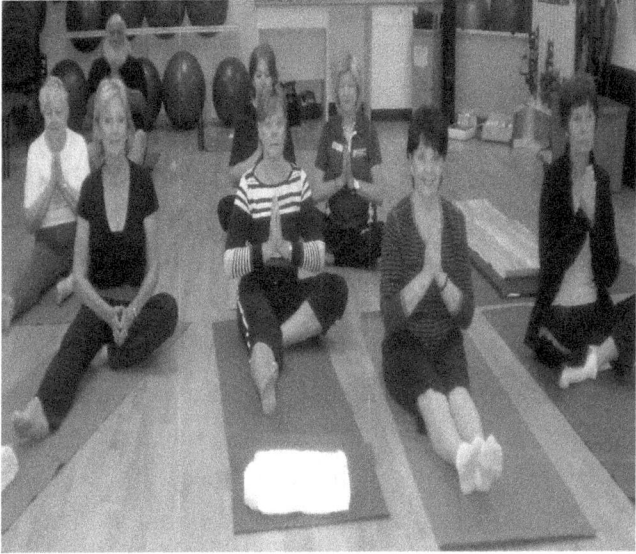

Chapter 8

How flexible are you?

There are a lot of flexibility benefits from practicing yoga. Studies have shown that long term immobilization of muscles and joints speed up the degenerative process causing further problems such as arthritis. If this is left untreated, it can further complicate into the loss of flexibility and strength.

As we age, simple tasks such as stretching, reaching and bending become a challenge. If you are unable to touch your toes, it is a good indication that you are losing flexibility. This can lead into a host of other restrictions and difficulties with every-day activities, such as;

- Getting out of bed
- Climbing stairs
- Getting in and out of vehicles
- Putting on your shoes or socks or tying your laces.
- Keeping up with others in a group
- Driving- turning your head to check your blind spot

- Fastening your clothing
- Not being able to be a participant in activities you enjoy

If you are experiencing any of these restrictions, it is time to do something about it. Start a yoga class and get moving for your own benefit and independence.

It is important to note that certain stretches or exercises may actually be harmful for people who are experiencing joint and muscle pain. This is why you will need to consult with a doctor or trained professional to find a program that is safe yet effective for your body. Become aware of your limitations and do not compound your problem in the name of exercise. Do whatever it takes to remain independent and well. It is your body that is striving to stay forever young by exercising. Reclaim your wellness.

Here are some of the benefits of yoga and why people choose yoga:
- Pulse rate decreases
- Respiratory rate decreases
- Blood Pressure decreases

- EEG – alpha brain waves increase (theta, delta, and beta waves also increase during various stages of meditation)
- Cardiovascular efficiency increases
- Respiratory efficiency increases
- Gastrointestinal function normalizes
- Endocrine function normalizes
- Excretory functions improve
- Musculoskeletal flexibility goes up
- Joint range of motion increases
- Grip strength increases
- Eye-hand coordination improves
- Dexterity skills improve
- Reaction time improves
- Posture improves
- Strength and resiliency increases
- Endurance increases
- Energy level increases
- Weight normalizes
- Sleep improves
- Immunity increases
- Pain decreases
- Depth perception improves
- Balance improves
- Integrated functioning of body parts improve

Psychological Benefits of Yoga
- Somatic and kinesthetic awareness increase
- Mood improves and subjective well-being increases
- Self-acceptance and self-actualization increase
- Social adjustment increases
- Anxiety and Depression decrease
- Hostility decreases
- Concentration /attention improves
- Memory improves
- Learning efficiency improves
- Self-actualization increases
- Social skills increase
- Depth perception improves

Biochemical Benefits of Yoga
- Glucose decreases
- Sodium decreases
- Total cholesterol decreases
- Triglycerides decrease
- HDL cholesterol increases
- LDL cholesterol decreases
- VLDL cholesterol decreases

- Cholinesterase increases
- Catecholamines decrease
- ATPase increases
- Hematocrit increases
- Hemoglobin increases
- Lymphocyte count increases
- Total white blood cell count decreases
- Thyroxin increases
- Vitamin C increases
- Total serum protein increases

PAGE 103

Chapter 9

What is Yoga Fusion?

Yoga fusion is yoga interpreted at an altered level. It is more of an attempt to include a number of other fitness exercises, such as Pilates, to the practice series of yoga poses offered in a basic yoga class. The fusion aspect may include strength training, resistance work, and cardiovascular activities, some elements of dance or Pilates moves. Most yoga fusion classes attempt to provide the versatility and challenges along with the breathing segment of yoga while also offering extensive toning, muscle-building or fat-burning activities.

The primary type of yoga fusion is yoga and Pilates sometimes referred to as Yogilates. Pilates is the work-out of singling out small muscle groups and doing subtle strength exercises that target those muscles. Pilates exercise is a good addition to the overall stretching and strengthening offered in yoga.

Another yoga fusion that has gained attention is booty ballet. It's a showy name for what is basically a full-body fitness class integrating stretches, poses, dance moves, balancing and breathing.

The advantages of most yoga fusion workouts are that they are energetic and stimulating yet attainable. They can offer the mental and spiritual benefits of yoga along with the physical benefits of a cardiovascular workout.

Trainers keep the pace invigorating and the movements interesting. As a result, there are fewer chances of boredom or fatigue. Most yoga fusion workouts can be adapted for people with various needs as well as for beginners.

Most yoga fusion workouts are a mixture of warm-up, stretching, breathing, centering, strength training, and cardiovascular conditioning along with flexibility work, typically accompanied by music. The main objective of Yogilates is to promote a quick and steady development of strength and definition of muscles.

Yoga fusion is available to people of all levels of fitness. However, the very beginners should probably take traditional yoga classes first. This is because yoga fusion has less concentration on framework and more focus on keeping the heart rate up.

What Is Chair Yoga?

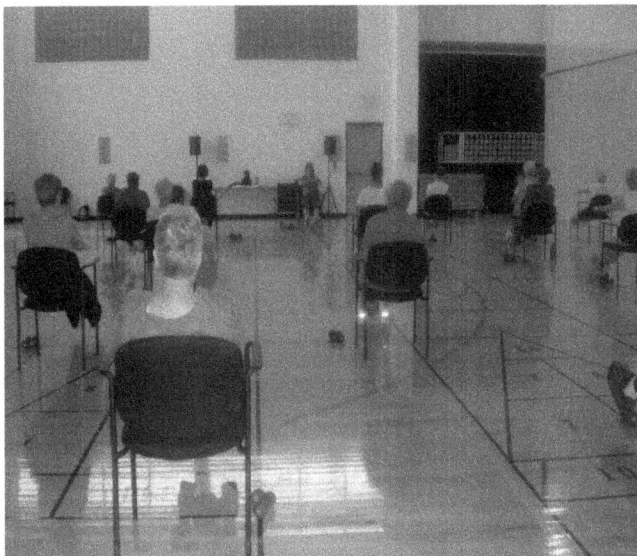

The defining characteristic of 'Chair Yoga' would be to say it is a gentle approach to yoga. This form of yoga is practiced while seated in a chair or the chair may be used as a prop for support, while standing. It does not have any acknowledgement as a distinct or unique discipline of yoga, like other traditional forms of yoga.

Most chair yoga classes use only a chair, eliminating the need for a mat all together. This reduces the difficulty of getting on and off the floor, which may be challenging for some people.

Chair yoga is best suitable for older people with restricted flexibility. However, it is also perfect for anyone with injuries who wants to keep practicing yoga.

Chair yoga, thought of as a gentler form of yoga, and uses a chair for additional support. Most of the exercises are done while seated, or standing while holding onto a chair. This is a great way to start yoga. This method for practicing yoga is made easy for people of all ages and those with limited mobility. A few seated positions can still build strength, increase circulation and the flow of oxygen. Remember any yoga is better than no yoga at all.

Success in yoga is not calculated by the level of ability to carry out a posture. Rather, it is done by a beneficial attitude and experiencing the benefits of doing the pose at a fitting level that best suits your needs and abilities.

Chapter 10

What is Pilates?

Pilates is a style of exercise that was developed by Joseph Pilates. He placed an emphasis on the balanced enhancement of the body through core strength, flexibility, and awareness which can be achieved through deliberate, competent, and smooth movements.

Pilates increases the flexibility of the spine, posture, breathing and alignment. It is believed that it "strengthens the core better than any exercise ever invented."

The important elements of Pilates consist of the placement of the breath in the ribs, articulating the spine, stabilizing the pelvis and shoulders for better balance, and the importance on linking movements together in a smooth and elegant way. This helps to develop the dexterity and concentration level. Even though the focus of Pilates is on flexibility, strength and balance, practitioners walk away with a long, lean and toned body.

Pilates is a unique method of exercise. Core strength is the foundation of Pilates exercise. The core muscles are the deep, internal muscles of the abdomen and back. When the core muscles are physically powerful in doing their job, as they are trained to do in Pilates, they work in harmony with the more superficial muscles of the body to support the spine and movement. This also helps to relieve back pain and strengthen the back muscles.

As you strengthen and build your core muscle you develop stability all the way through your entire torso. This is one of the ways Pilates helps people cope with back pain. As the body is properly supported, pressure on the back is relieved and the body can move freely and effectively and with less pain.

The six Pilates principles are centering, control, flow, breath, precision, and concentration. They are the essential ingredients in an expert quality Pilates workout. The Pilates approach has always put emphasis on quality over quantity, and you will find that, unlike many other systems of exercise, Pilates exercises do not include a lot of repetitions for each move. Instead, you will do each exercise fully, with precision movements to obtain considerable results in a shorter amount of time than one would ever imagine.

Core strength and torso steadiness, along with the six Pilates principles, set the Pilates method apart from many other types of exercise. Weight lifting, for example, can put a lot of awareness on arm or leg strength without paying any consideration to the fact that those limbs are joined to the rest of the body! At the end of the day, those who are able to do well at their sport learn to use their core muscles. However, in Pilates this integrative approach is essential and taught from the beginning.

Mat Work and Equipment
Pilates exercises are done either on a mat on the floor with or on exercise equipment developed by Joseph Pilates. The exercise equipment that is used for Pilates usually makes use of pulleys and resistance from your own body weight on the machine and graduated levels of springs. Mats are probably the best-known piece of equipment that you will encounter at a Pilates studio.

It is not like the customary fitness programs that fatigue the muscles and can cause injuries due to excessive use. Pilates is a holistic form of whole body training that leaves you feeling invigorated and lively with a feeling of physical and mental well-being.

With regular practice, Pilates can:
- Increase balance between strength and flexibility, in particularly the core and back muscles
- Improves posture, balance, and core strength
- Improves co-ordination, stability, and posture awareness
- Improves bone density and joint health
- Increases lung capacity and circulation
- Releases stress
- Promotes injury prevention
- Improves performance technique for athletes and dancers

Chapter 11

What is Nia?

The Nia Technique is Fusion Fitness at Its Best!It is a stimulating blend of dance arts, martial arts and healing arts. It is the first and the most superior form of combination fitness. It combines healing, dance and martial arts into the ultimate "East meets West" technique to tone your body, mind, and spirit. Nia is sometimes referred to as "aerobic yoga," and is a path to condition, heal and express yourself through movement and awareness.

Pilates blend elements of dance, Tai Chi, martial arts, and yoga. It is a contemplative physical practice that appeals to those who embrace creativity and flexibility in a wellness program. Balancing technical exactness with free-form expression, Nia brings the body, mind, emotions and spirit to optimum health through music, movement and self-expression, guided by the sensation of pleasure.

This cardiovascular program uses the whole-body, in addition to exuberance, grounded movement, and is flexible to every level of fitness. It is suitable for every age and all body types, even those with special restrictions.

This combination creates a joint action that no out-of-the-way technique can match. Nia's new creative idea of replacing punishment with pleasure preaches about doing things the easy way instead of the hard way. Nia is designed for anybody. It is ageless and limitless, complete and effective for every person everywhere. This also applies to many professionals like athletes, dancers, and fitness instructors. It can also be done by children, special needs groups and the elderly. This discipline adheres to the philosophy; if it feels right, just keep doing it.

While delivering cardiovascular benefits and whole-body conditioning, Nia creates a loving relationship with one's own body by tuning into the Body's own technique: the instinctive intelligence of the body. Through Nia's exercises, you learn to cultivate an awareness of your life through physical consciousness, allowing the language of the Body to direct your actions and choices, leading to a general state of what Nia calls "Dynamic Ease."

Done barefoot to music, each person is encouraged to move at his or her own level of intensity, adapting the fifty two moves to their body potential at any given moment.

Nia is a personal growth, body-mind-spirit fitness program. It is a "living system" that performs with the innate wisdom and brainpower of the body, mind, spirit, and emotions. It supports the "Pleasure Principle." If the movement fits the body, and you feel no discomfort, keep on doing it, if it hurts, stop!

Nia touches people emotionally, in their hearts, inspiring them to get fit and healthy by creating a deep personal desire to explore their potential and love their growth. Fitness, health, well-being, and self-love are a genuine result from the Nia experience. Nia provides power to all, students and teachers alike, to create their own movement options by offering students a flexible structure. It is up to the individual person to do modifications to suit their needs.

What makes Nia so innovative is its unlimited adaptability. Everyone can do Nia! There are three levels of intensity for every movement that is provided. This is done in a variety and a range of motions to create a very user-friendly fitness experience. Starting with athletes to dancers to those who are just making a return into fitness, students of all levels and backgrounds will be challenged and energized.

To allow for improved strength and more pleasure of movement, Nia is always done barefoot. Participants wear loose-fitting comfy layers of clothes which they can shed as they warm up.

A typical class begins with flowing stretches. There is a relaxing ebb and flow to the amount of force required as the pace gently increases toward a low-impact cardio workout of swifter whole-body movements. Self-consciousness plays a vital role; those who adjust their level of movement according to their body's response will benefit most. After 40 minutes into a session, the tempo gradually changes to more blended poses and luxurious stretches. Some Nia teachers employ soothingly guided relaxation to quiet the minds and bodies of everyone present as the session comes to a close.

Remember to ask yourself the following questions. Are you giving your heart a real workout while you are burning fat and calories and building your muscles all at the same time. This is a good question to start with. There is no need for pounding, running or panting. You are swaying your body to the music; to a rhythm that is alluring to you. You are smiling and having fun. Your mind is calm, and your body is fluid. This is Nia!

To really get a feel for Nia, you need to pay attention to the continual changing background of music that plays during a Nia class. This is truly unique unlike the music of other fitness groups. A well adapted soundtrack is the most important yarn that interlaces the basics of Nia together and makes classes different, unpredictable, and enjoyable. Participants might enjoy several varieties during one class: Harmonious, melodious and rhythmic and anything in between, as each musical passage stimulates the senses and the body in different ways.

They are a diverse group; not everyone practices Nia for the same reasons. While some use Nia as a source of healthy pursuit while others use Nia as a place to find inner peace.

Many community classes are a testament where one can witness a wonderful cross-section of younger and older participants taking part in a shared fitness activity. Some of the participants may include grandparents with newly replaced hips and others come to rehabilitate knees and stiff joints. Younger, more toned participants are keen to sustain or test personal fitness levels. The younger and the older, perspire, breathe, and laugh together. While sharing their Nia fitness routine at the same time, they demonstrate a healthy zest for life. They are having fun!

Nia is a contentment centered fitness program that will not only get you in fantastic shape, it will completely change how you feel about your body and exercise. Nia is pleasurable and fun! People of all ages and walks of life are attracted to Nia. Done regularly, Nia can show you the way to a healthier physical outlook and a comfortable, more enjoyable daily living. Most importantly, Nia is invigorating and fun! Nia stimulates people and that keeps them coming back. It is not just for the physical benefits, but in part because of the way their lives change after they start practicing Nia.

Chapter 12

What is Barefoot Dancing?

Many ancient cultures, such as the African, Egyptian, Indian, and Greek, saw very little need for footwear, and most of the time, preferred to go barefoot. Bare feet are also seen as a sign of humility and reverence, and many religions embrace being barefoot. They remove their shoes as a sign of respect towards someone of a higher standing than themselves. Bare foot dancing has always existed and will continue to grow and obtain more participants till the end of time.

The Romans wore clothes and shoes as a status symbol to show their power and standing in society. On the other hand, their peasants and slaves remained barefoot. Remember the invention of shoes is a lot more recent. Moving barefoot also results in a more natural gait, allowing for additional rocking motion of the foot, eliminating the hard heel strike and causing fewer collision forces in the foot and lower leg.

There are many sports people who partake in barefoot activities, such as hiking, running, water skiing, beach volleyball, gymnastics, martial arts, swimming, surfing, and water polo. So go ahead and shed the shoes. It also allows your feet to breathe after all and the babies love it.

Many people and cultures prefer to go barefoot occasionally, often, or everywhere, and they are known as a bare footer. In most instances, it is usually a voluntary choice, as the person enjoys being barefoot, in contrast to someone who cannot afford shoes.

There is also hula or Hawaiian dance, African dance, belly dance, folk dance, hoop dance and cardio hoop dance. Barefoot dancing is called by other names, such as freestyle dance, barefoot boogie, free dance, freestyle dance, dance jam, and dance church. They can be done anywhere but here in North America it is held in dance studios where there are spaces with open areas and wood floors to allow for the flow of movement. It has entered our society once again in some of the more modern dance styles such as, "So you think you can dance," and even on "Dancing with the stars".

When you enter a barefoot dance studio, you will become aware of a number of things happening in the room. First, you will notice a wide range of ages among the participants, from toddlers up through great-grandpas and grandmas. It is a relatively safe environment. It is evident that they are all there for the same reason. You will notice the lights are dimmed so that you may dance without self-consciousness. There will likely be relaxing cushions scattered around the borders of the dance space for people to unwind. There is absolutely no need to be shy because everyone will be dancing barefoot! You will notice a compassionate approach of respect and humbleness among the members. Some barefoot dancing groups may have accessories for movement, such as large exercise balls, hula hoops, and light streamers.

Even though people do not dance with partners as in ballroom dance, sometimes participants at barefoot dance sessions participate in a special dance form that makes contact with each other as if to draw strength from their energy. This form of dancing begins with each dancer, touching another dancer at a point of body contact, which changes continuously as the dancing proceeds. Some dancers may leap and roll as they progress, while remaining respectful and careful of other dancers on the floor, while other dancers may move slowly and gracefully while moving on the floor.

African dancing is very energetic and playful. It can be viewed as a playground for connection and Self Expression. Many individuals come together in an open space and with bare feet. The participants move around enjoying the elated feeling of moving their body freely through space and time. Tribal dance is a dynamic self-guided spiritual movement practice where people move, play, connect, sweat, stretch, sound, unwind, renew, release, contact, and improvise. In the end, you transform yourself because you feel free from being judged for your co-ordination and style. In barefoot dancing, anything goes. There is no need to feel intimidated and judged. Be free spirited and enjoy your dance after all no matter what you do, or how you do it, you are moving. You are exercising and that is a good thing for the body, mind and spirit. Barefoot dancing can even be seen on television.

Chapter 13

Aquafit Aquarobics Water Aerobics Swimming

There are so many great things to respect when considering aquatic exercise.   Aerobics in the water is more challenging than on land because there is constant resistance from the water so you are always working harder.   The buoyancy of the water, however, allows you to feel and believe that you're working less.   Each person is able to keep their own intensity unlike land sessions where you feel it is necessary to keep up with the instructor, and most of the body is hidden so people feel less awkward.   Participants feel safe in the water as they cannot fall and hurt themselves. It is possible to work multiple muscles at the same time or you can isolate specific muscles.

Remember, you might not feel like you're working too hard so you don't get caught overdoing it. Start out slowly, at least for your first few classes until you know what to expect and how your body reacts in the water.

Positive Effects of Buoyancy: Buoyancy in water decreases the amount of shock which is transmitted through the bones, joints and ligaments upon landing. It decreases the effect of gravity. Special needs participants including the obese, the elderly who may have fragile bones, the arthritic, the disabled, the injured athlete, as well as pre- or post natal women will exercise in a relative comfort zone and with ease in the water.

Decreased gravity results in decreased joint loading. This permits improved range of joint mobility which provides a resistance to joint injury. The force of buoyancy assists venous return. On land, the downward forces of gravity push the blood toward the feet. The cardiovascular system works against gravity to take blood to the heart. In the water, the upward rise of buoyancy counteracts the downward pull of gravity, thus assisting venous return. This can be a factor to lower exercise heart rates during aqua-fitness.

Positive Effects of Hydrostatic Pressure: Venous return and cardiac functions are greatly enhanced by hydrostatic pressure. Hydrostatic pressure helps participants to exercise more vigorously with less stress on the cardiovascular system and produces a reduced training heart rate for a given workload. Hydrostatic pressure reduces swelling in the tissue of injured or edematous (swollen) joints or limbs below the water. The pressure of water on the chest wall creates a training effect for the respirator muscles.

Positive Effects of Turbulence: Currents and eddies in the water massage the skin, promoting circulation and relaxation. Turbulence plays a role in the resistance felt in aquatic exercise. The core muscles are trained to become stronger as participants learn to steady their bodies against turbulence. Exercises can be designed to work with or against turbulence, thereby increasing or decreasing intensity.

Positive Effects of Thermal Conductivity: The water 'wicks' away excess body heat during exercise creating a cooler, more comfortable workout. Blood that would be shunted to the skin for cooling is then available to the working muscles. The heart does not have to work as hard if the body stays cool. Pool temperatures can be adjusted to meet all specials needs groups such as those suffering from arthritis or rehabilitation (30 to 38 degrees Celsius) or intense athletic training around 27 degrees Celsius. Studies have shown that with regular water exercise there is a noteworthy increase in muscular strength and endurance level, flexibility, cardio respiratory conditioning, and decreased body fat. Besides the physical advantages, there are mood improvements. People adapt a positive attitude and feel better about themselves while obtaining more knowledge on the workings of their body.

The participants are able to defy their nervous and respiratory systems by way of the magical properties of water. By way of enjoying the benefits of balance, agility, coordination and endurance, they are better able to be in control of their independence and their everyday living. Water resistance is the perfect work setting for strength-training. By employing the water's resistance rather than equipment, the body receives an all over toning while working on isolated and/or corresponding muscles groups. The water's buoyancy reduces the joint impact. During the summer months, we are less inclined to get involved in fitness activities as a result of the heat. However, you can definitely carry out your workout in a pool that is comfortable, refreshing, and healthy. Aqua-fitness is an exercise for everyone regardless of their limitations.

Chapter 14

Other Options

Well, that covers most kinds of classes but what about the other options? Hiring a personal trainer will offer you even more opportunities to change your body. A trainer will be available to you either in your gym or even at your own home or office. Personal trainers train you, personally, beginning with an assessment of your overall fitness level.

The trainer will develop a training program specifically for you, based on your body's abilities, current fitness level and your fitness goals. Your trainer will demonstrate each exercise for you and spot you as you execute these movements, ensuring you stay safe and comfortable throughout your routine. Some trainers work out of a gym or studio and will meet with you at the gym at your convenience. They can help you become acquainted with the equipment and machines that have been intimidating you since you arrived. With the help of a trainer, you'll own those machines before you know it.

Some trainers will come to your house and train you using objects or equipment you have at home. They will try to accommodate your schedule. You can arrange for them to arrive at your most productive time of day to ensure you work hard and get a lot done. If necessary, they will bring their own tools that they may loan to you or bring to you, depending how often you meet. This is more costly, of course, but if you're a busy person it could be worthwhile to know that you could see a trainer at 6am, 3 times a week, in the comfort of your own home.

Some people hire a trainer on a regular basis, meeting daily, weekly or monthly to update, motivate, and make changes to their program. In addition to instruction on proper technique, your trainer might keep a log of your progress, making changes as he or she sees necessary. This one-on-one method is a great way to stay motivated and stimulated throughout your fitness program.

Fitness Tools

Your trainer will likely have a bag of fitness tools that might look like both toys and torture devices. These items are simply portable methods to replicate working with weights or weight machines without the heavy bulk and weight. Most of these tools are available to the general public but before you bring them all home, let's find out what they're for and how they're used.

SKIPPING ROPE

If you're like most people, the words "skipping rope" remind you of your childhood and school days. However, nowadays, jumping rope is much more than child's play. It offers a great cardiovascular workout, strengthens bones and burns calories and helps to feel young and in control.

Skipping helps with co ordination and to keeps you light on your toes. It is good for timing and coordination. It also functions as a very efficient fat burner thus making it one of the most favorite types of aerobic exercise among boxers.

One of the best things about skipping is that you have to invest very little money to get started. All you need are a comfortable pair of shoes and a rope. Get yourself a rope that is light-weight with foam grips to help prevent it from slipping out of your hands.

To know if your rope is the right length, stand in the middle of the rope. The handles of the rope should reach up to your armpits.

Jumping Tips:

- The surface you choose to jump on will affect your workout. Jump on a wood floor or rubber mat, because those surfaces absorb shock. Stay away from concrete.

- Turn the rope with your wrists while keeping your hands at waist level.

- Keep your back straight and your head up.

- Make your jumps low, like a boxer.

- Build up your endurance slowly, but aim to jump for five to 10 minutes three or four times per week.

FREE WEIGHTS

These are handheld dumbbells that range from 1 to 100 lbs. They are commonly used to challenge muscle strength and endurance.

When you use free weights, your muscles are completely engaged as you lift and lower the weight.   You also have to balance the weights in your hands to ensure proper form and motion. Proper form is crucial to a safe injury-free workout.

STABILITY BALL SWISS BALL RESIST-A-BALL

The stability ball was originally introduced for use in the therapy of patients with neurological disorders and spinal injuries.   Leading the way was Mike and Stephanie Morris in the 1990s. Resist-A-Ball crossed over into the fitness arena and is an essential piece of training equipment for nearly every personal trainer and fitness professional.   The thing that makes the stability ball so useful in fitness is its instability!   The challenge of an unstable surface triggers your stabilizer muscles, which help with overall balance and stability.   This ball is a great tool to use to improve your balance and stability, as well as challenge your body in a different way.

Don't let the instability factor scare you away from the fitness ball.   If you sit properly on the ball you won't have to worry about falling.

Begin by finding the right ball for you.   General rule of thumb, when you're sitting on the ball, your hip should be level with the tops of your knees. Make sure your feet stay under, or beyond your knees when you are on the ball, not under the ball itself. Also, sit on the "front" half of the ball, never on the "peak".

Finally, make a nice wide stance to increase your base of support. That's the area of ground you cover. The bigger your base of support, the more stable you will be. As your stabilizer muscle groups get stronger and you become more used to this unstable seat, you will be able to challenge your body by changing your stance to a narrow or one-legged stance.

This ball is used for a variety of exercises in both a seated and lying down position. You can work with weights for resistance exercises, use your own body weight, or even use the ball for resistance. Have your trainer help you feel comfortable on the ball and show all the exercise options available on the ball. The stability ball will add difficulty to your work. Even when you're just sitting on it you're engaging underused muscles.

RESISTANCE TUBING – DYNABANDS

The main difference between tubing and free weights is that there is no easy part of the movement. Resistance is continuous in both the lifting and the lowering part of the exercise which challenges your muscles in a different way. The bands provide smooth resistance through the entire range of motion.

Resistance band training is especially ideal for people who travel as this tool will fit in a suitcase or even a hand bag. This is great because it is ready to go anywhere, but it's also great for small spaces where there is not enough room for a big piece of equipment. In spite of its small size, it is a huge tool with hundreds of different exercises you can perform for the upper body, lower body, and core, especially when you add a door attachment.

You can work your arms, legs, back, chest, and abs by using these bands in many different ways. Some bands have handles attached, while others are band-only which is a little more uncomfortable to hold. Never wrap the bands around your hands as this will interfere with circulation and overall comfort. Also, remember not to squeeze the band or handle too tightly as this will engage your forearm muscles unnecessarily.

KETTLEBELLS

Kettlebells are like cannonballs with a looped handle and they are a different kind of dumbbell. They range in weight from 2 to 100 lbs. They have been used for centuries, but the origin is obscure. Many assume that this form of weight training was developed in Russia during the time of the Cold War. Others believe the use of heavy round weights actually originated as part of the Scottish Highland sporting culture using curling stones as the principal model.

Weight training with kettlebells affect many muscle groups and stretches the body across a wide range of motion. They can work well with any training program, but these weights are more cumbersome than traditional dumbbells and are more challenging to control. Like anything new, it takes practice. Your forearms work harder with kettlebells than with regular dumbbell weights because you have to stabilize the bell in your grip and hold them firmly.

Keep in mind that you are working with a weight. If you are concerned about hitting your forearms, special forearm guards are available. As with any new program, speak with a professional who is familiar with this style of training. Do not over-train. Be sure to rest your muscles for at least a day between kettlebell sessions.

YOGA BLOCKS & BANDS

Under normal circumstances yoga equipment, tools, and props may not be needed when practicing yoga but they have always been useful aids to practitioners. Be warned, that it is most important to feel relaxed and comfortable when doing the poses. Most yoga tools are intended to provide extra support to help you get deeper into a pose or do the pose better.

Yoga Mats: The yoga mat is probably the most important tool for yoga as it acts as cushioning between you and the ground or floor. It also gives you more traction for hands and feet which prevents slipping while trying to perform asanas.

Yoga Blocks: Yoga blocks are roughly nine inches long, six inches wide, and either three or four inches high. The size of the yoga blocks is important, since students use them at each of their various heights. Standing on the skinny end will allow you to stretch up an extra nine inches. The flat three-inch edge enables you to stand up six inches while the six-inch plane gives you a smaller lift. While we often only use one block at a time, it is useful to have two matching blocks for many beginner poses. Using blocks will help take the pressure off the arms and upper body muscles when executing some postures by building up the floor so you can reach down to it.

Yoga Straps: One reason people stay away from practicing yoga is that they think they are not flexible enough. Yoga is not about showing off how flexible you are but about strengthening your body and your spine in all directions with the goal of creating a union between the body, mind and spirit. All that matters is for you to try to perform the pose the right way without pushing yourself too far. By practicing yoga you will develop flexibility, strength, and become more energetic.

The yoga strap which is decidedly helpful for beginners may be made of cotton or nylon. These straps help you stretch out deeper or hold a pose longer. Yoga straps are particularly useful in bound poses if your hands cannot reach each other, or for poses where you need to hold your foot but cannot reach it. It can help you to hold stretches and postures.

Overall, it is important to keep your body "thinking" about what you're asking of it. Changing up exercise routines is essential to progress. If you only ever lift 5 pound weights then you'll only be able to lift 5 pounds or less. The body needs to be challenged in order to change and changing up exercises will keep your brain working and keep you from getting bored.

Enjoy your journey. It will be wonderful, and you never know what you'll find out about yourself, your body, and what new things you'll learn. It's all so exciting so keep learning, keep moving, and don't forget to keep breathing.

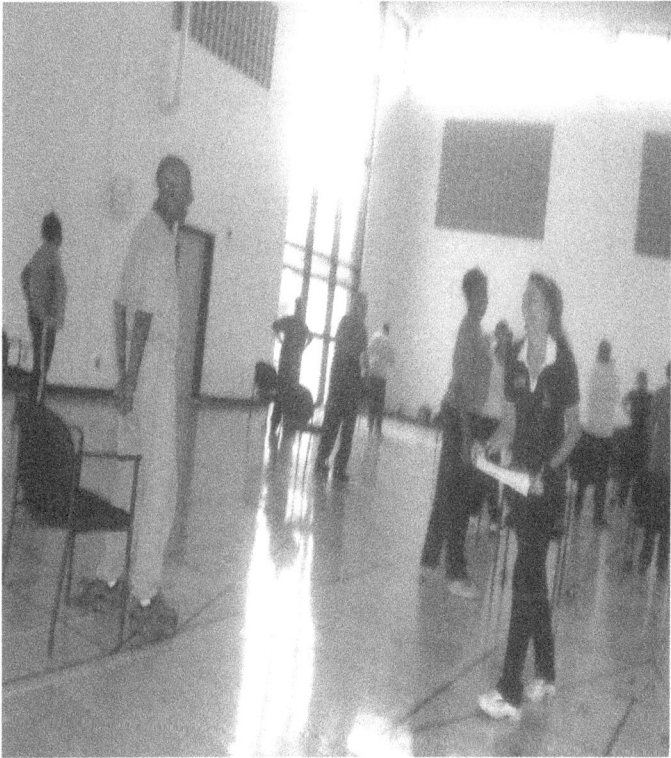

Chapter 15

The Fun Side of Being a Senior

Well, we have certainly discussed some of the different exercises that are available to you. We looked at how they are and also what is involved in participating in these exercises. We have examined the various pitfalls of over exercising why it is important to consider them before starting an exercise regime. However, we also explored how fun it can be to get involved while still benefiting and experiencing great satisfaction.

How about getting involved as a volunteer that will actually allow you to see the benefits of both sides? Think about getting involved in a foster a grandparent programme. There is so much to gain, for example, it would give you an opportunity to share your past knowledge, especially if you had a special skill. A young person listens more intently to a grandparent than a parent.

What Is The Foster Grandparent Program?

The Foster Grandparent Program is an unpaid assistant program that offers seniors age 60 and older a paid non-taxable stipend to serve as mentors, tutors and caregivers for children and youth with special needs. As foster grandparents, you can set your own hours per week in community-based organizations such as elementary schools, youth detention centers, parent-child centers, hospitals, day care programs, drug treatment facilities, correctional institutions, shelters, early childhood programs, after-school programs and I am sure there are many other areas where your service is needed like in a special needs home. Involvement in such a programme would also mean that you must love children and be willing to devote twenty hours a week.

So just how does it helps a student?

Foster grandparents tutor elementary school students to assist other students to learn better reading skills. It also provides poignant support to children who have had the misfortune of being abused and neglected. You are also presented with the opportunity to mentor troubled teenagers and young mothers as well as care for infants and children with physical and developmental disabilities. In the process, they enrich our communities by providing youth services that a community budget does not allow for and it bridges the gap between generations.

This might cause you to question how you benefit from such a program.

With a lifetime of knowledge of having raised their own children and a willingness to become vulnerable and reach out to someone in need, foster grandparents have much to offer to a lost young person. In some cases, foster grandparents receive a modest tax-free stipend, reimbursement for transportation, a daily meal during service, an annual physical examination, and accident and liability insurance while on duty. In addition to these benefits, the program provide participants with the opportunity to share a lifetime of experience with youths, and join many Canadians and Americans who are strengthening communities across the country as members of the National Senior Service Corps.

For some families, grandparents are the ties that bind a family together. However, that blood-bond isn't there for every child. The nurturing offered by foster grandparents helps children to rise above their unfortunate life in their physical, psychological, educational and social development, and to acquire a better self image.

When older people invest their care and love, children can benefit a sense of values and coping skills to help them respond to life's challenges. In fact, studies indicate that volunteering enhances one's physical, mental and social well being and enriches the quality of life for the volunteer. Some of your duties might involve the following:

Help students with homework assignments. Check that they are complete and submitted on time. Students sometimes find that their foster grandparent is much more approachable and less intimidating. They tend to think of the foster grandparent as a friend.

Support students in their reading, and writing activities. Work in small groups and/or one on one sharing your love of books. Help students with journal activities. Teaching and guiding them to learn about the essentials of life will support their development skills that are necessary later on in life. Teaching them to be faithful and diligent in completing small chores will help them to be a more responsible citizen in their futures.

Volunteers who work with infants provide them with a nurturing experience that only a "Grandparent" can give. The warmth of your hugs and cuddles help them to feel more loved and secure because they have a shoulder to lean on. Tell them stories and read to them.

If you enjoy math and have the skills, then share your passion for math or science with students by being an instructor or classroom partner in these subjects. Math will help them in everyday life when dealing with financial issues.

It is of great advantage for a senior to lend a hand in general classroom activities that demands your own special talents and interests. This can be achieved simply by being a positive influence to the children.

Share your love of arts and crafts and/or music with students through activities that address these areas of interest. Just knowing that the student has a caring listener can make all the difference in their progress.

If you don't like working with children then there are so many other avenues to explore such as:

The local theatre where you can support them with duties such as setting up props, stage help, ticket sales, seating patrons and even helping with the mail that would need to be sent out to the seasonal ticket holder and even helping with phone calls. By involving yourself with young people, it helps you to keep feeling young. You laugh a lot and indulge yourself in the fun and games.

If you are a Gardener, volunteer in a nursery or garden centre. On the other hand, you can also work in a bingo hall by passing out bingo cards and being a runner.

If you have always wanted to learn photography, here is your chance to take a course and learn how. Then you can go on trips to take pictures of beautiful scenery and go home to make a painting of it. Take portraits of your family and make up albums as gifts. Do mini videos of special events and give it as a keepsake is another hobby that may interest you.

How about volunteering at your local seniors centre? You can use your time teaching others some of your skills. Included in these skills are art, games, music, and computers and some of the programs such as word, excel, internet, face book and file management. As you teach these skills, you will realize how open you are to embracing new skills. In the end, your grandchildren and other loved ones will be so impressed with you keeping up with the changing times.

If you are an artistic person who likes working with your hands, teach sewing, cooking, painting, carving, and embroidery like bunka, crewel and needlepoint. If you are a painter, try teaching oil painting, acrylic painting and roughing. You can even try your hand at making something of beauty such as tatting, plastic canvas, Jewelry and teddy bear making for the grandchildren as gifts. There's also ceramics. You might want to try your hand at making some heirloom pieces for your family as gifts.

If you are a Dancer, try teaching other seniors to line dance, ballroom dance, clogging, hula, square dance or whatever type dance you are skilful in.

If you are a great organizer and like to plan, why not try getting involved in planning road trips for the seniors, or an afternoon of high tea or even summer walking tours to see local gardens.

Organize a treasure hunt for the children and board games and make sure to include a group that will listen to electronic books. It is important to remember that children have different likes and dislikes. You just need to tap into their interests and create activities that will best serve their needs. You can even try your hand at organizing a choir. Plan bus tours to the casino and the races; however, you should caution your group to take only the amount of money with them that they can afford to lose. Exercise self control at all times, have fun but do not allow anyone to become broke having fun because it is no longer fun. Be sure to leave all credit and bank cards at home to resist the temptation of overspending.

If you have a passion for reading, you can volunteer to read at your local library. You can read to children in the summer months, or to seniors who love books but can no longer see to read.

Enjoy meeting new people! How about working with welcome wagon or helping new immigrants settle in their new city and showing them the ropes of getting around on the bus or how to find a business they might be looking for. Since you speak English, teach the new immigrant to speak English if their mother tongue is another language. Help them to get over the culture shock. Teach them how to earn their citizenship and become a citizen that will enhance your county.

If you enjoy writing, try joining a writing group and write your memoirs and leave a written legacy for your grandchildren. Help them to learn about your childhood and what it was like. Write about the childhood stories you were told.

Get together with a group and watch classic movies, like the old John Wayne movies or Agatha Christie mysteries. It's great to watch those epic movies from bygone days, and many of them are available to buy or rent online or from your local video store.

If you have a bucket list, write it down and work toward accomplishing every last one of them. The one beautiful thing is, at your age nothing is forbidden.

If all the above is not of any interest, then you can join a group and play fun games such as shuffle board, lawn bowling, carpet bowling, badminton, ping pong, volleyball and golf. Then there are board games such as chess, checkers, backgammon, mahjong or cards such as bridge and Euchre. Try learning to play dominoes too.

Should you decide to stay on working part time, and you love the game of golf try getting a job at a local course. If you enjoy golfing, there couldn't be a better place to work. There are many job openings at courses and country clubs including Golf Course Ranger, Golf Course/Cart Maintenance, Food Service, Sales (in the Pro Shop) and Promotions/Marketing. Many golf courses offer employee incentives, and some even allow free use of the golf course. This is an excellent opportunity if you like to golf a lot.

Are you someone who would rather be busy volunteering at the local food bank and shelter? Become a member of the senior committee and have your say in what goes on in the centre. You will certainly enjoy having a voice on all the activities and what goes on at the centre.

What about if you love water and sailing? You can take advantage of your Marina expertise. If you love the water, why not give your time volunteering at a marina. Marinas has several openings for Boat Cleaners, Fuel Attendants and

Harbormasters/ Managers. Some of the more busy marinas may also have a need for Boat Instructors and Tour Guides. In North America, marina jobs are usually seasonal which will allow you time to be a snow bird.

One of the biggest challenges you are most likely to face on retiring is maintaining the agility of your mind; making sure you keep your brain active. Volunteering to read to others in nursing homes could surely achieve that purpose, as well as help you relax. Moreover, it also offers you a cheap form of entertainment. So, why don't you join a good library or a book club and meet once a month to discuss the book and how the content made you feel? Critique the books and learn how opinion varies from one person to another. To make it even more fun the group should plan a meal to go with the discussion.

Feeling that you still want that degree that you had no time to earn? Register at a nearby university and pursue the degree you always desired. You will find that most universities will accept seniors into their program of choice for no fees. Nobody is too old to enroll for a course and it will certainly stimulate your mind and brain.

Or maybe you just feel like you want to learn more about investments and the stock market! Well, enroll in a financial course and learn how to manage and grow your investments. This is sure to impress your grandchildren because they will be coming to you for advice before long.

Enjoy driving? Try volunteering for Meal on wheels, you will be amazed how many wonderful shut ins you will meet that look forward to your visit each day. You are probably the only visitor they will have that day. It will make your day knowing you have made someone else's day a little brighter.

If you love animals then you already know how much joy a four-legged furry friend brings to your life. And if you do not quite fancy dogs, you could consider keeping other pets like a ferret, bird or cat. If you feel that you cannot afford to have a pet, then you can start a business of walking dogs or taking care of animals for vacationers.

Whatever you choose to do, make sure you keep a day timer and keep yourself busy. However, do not make yourself too busy that you have no down time for yourself. By keeping a day timer, it helps you to stay on track with all you would like to accomplish, and you will never be bored.

One of the upsides to this new involvement means you will meet a whole new bunch of friends with various interests. Be careful, your social calendar is apt to become quite full. You will meet some most interesting people with wonderful skills to offer.

Chapter 16

Basic Exercises for Major Muscle Groups

Perform 3 times per week, non-consecutive days

Squat

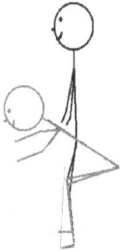

- As with all standing exercises, keep your knees soft, tummy tight and your shoulders down from your ears.
- Squat down, keeping your knees behind your toes.
- Push your butt back toward the wall behind you.
- Keep your spine long and always breathe.

Lunge

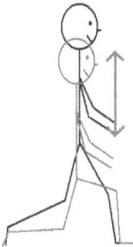

- Keep your front knee aligned above your heel, do not let knee roll forward.
- Keep body tall and aligned, with a straight line travelling from your back knee up through your hips and spine to the top of your head.
- Move your body down (for four counts) and up (for four counts), NOT forward and back.

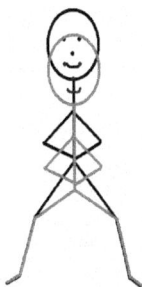

Plie

- Stand with feet wide, toes and knees pointing out to the corners.

- Move body down and up, keeping your body tall and erect

- Lie down on a mat or blanket on the floor with knees bent.

- Push hips up toward the ceiling keeping elbows and shoulders on the floor.

Hip Raises

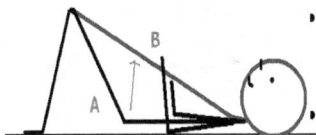

- For a greater challenge take your elbows off the floor.

- Lie on one side, hips stacked one above the other, top leg straight, bottom leg bent for balance.

Side Lying Leg Abduction

- Lift and lower top leg, keeping foot parallel to the floor throughout the entire movement.

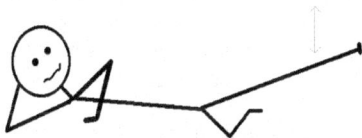

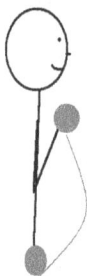

Bicep Curl

- Keep elbows connected to your body.

- Bend elbow to bring weight toward shoulder.

- Slowly straighten arm to beginning position.

- Keep back of wrist flat, do not fold hand backward.

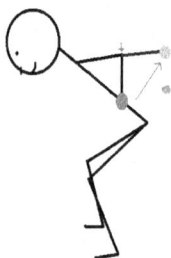

Tricep Kickback

Stand in a forward leaning position, bending at the hip, keeping spine tall and straight.

Lift elbows up behind you and isolate that position.

Slowly straighten and bend the arm to work the muscles on the back of the upper arm.

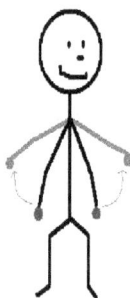

Lateral Raise

Stand tall with knees bent, tummy tight, and shoulders away from your ears.

Slowly lift weights up to the side, just to shoulder height.

Lower weights slowly to start position.

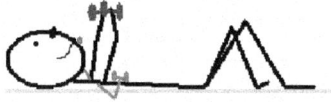

Chest Press on Mat

- Lie on your back on a mat or blanket on the floor, arms out to the side.

- Lift weights up toward ceiling, bringing them close but not together.

- Slowly lower arms toward floor.

Other books by this Author Norma Jean are:

1- Fables and Tales of Guyana Volume 1

2- Fables and Tales of Guyana Volume 2

3- Adventures of a Guyanese son Dennis

4- Macaw tell a history Story (History of   Guyana)

5- Folklores and Legends of Guyana

6- Memories and Reflection of life in Guyana

7- Anansi the Trickster Volume 1

8- Anansi the Trickster Volume 2

9- Anansi the Trickster Volume 3

10- Anansi the Trickster Volume 4

11- Anansi the Trickster Volume 5

12- Anansi the Trickster Volume 6

13- Anansi the Trickster Volume 7

14- Anansi the Trickster Volume 8

15- Anansi the Trickster Volume 9.

16- Anansi the Trickster Volume 10

17- First Nations legends and Folklore Volume 1

18- First Nations legends and Folklore Volume 2

19- Seniors Stay Forever young

20- Bubbles you are special Volume 1 (Exploring the living seas)

Please visit our website at www.childrensstories.ca

www.ingramcontent.com/pod-product-compliance
Lightning Source LLC
Chambersburg PA
CBHW072251270326
41930CB00010B/2345